# THE FACTS ABOUT ARTHRITIS

DID YOU KNOW:

- The term "arthritis" ............................... ns. The symptoms of ma .......................... no apparent reason

- 37 million people suffer from arthritis in one form or another

- Crippling can be avoided, reduced, or even overcome by innovative surgery

- Certain occupations and/or hobbies may make you more vulnerable to arthritic disease.

All the information you need—the sources, resources, and news of the very latest treatments—to give yourself

## RELIEF FROM
## CHRONIC ARTHRITIS PAIN

THE DELL MEDICAL LIBRARY

Relief from

# CHRONIC ARTHRITIS PAIN

Helene MacLean

*Foreword by Richard Wagman, M.D.*

A LYNN SONBERG BOOK

Correct diagnosis of the cause of pain and the proper course of treatment are matters that require individual attention from a physician. In addition, joint-pain can be a symptom of illnesses other than arthritis that would not respond to the methods described in this book. Any person who suffers joint-pain should therefore consult a physician before beginning any course of treatment.

Published by
Dell Publishing
a division of
Bantam Doubleday Dell Publishing Group, Inc.
666 Fifth Avenue
New York, New York 10103

Copyright © 1990 by Lynn Sonberg Book Services

Published by arrangement with Lynn Sonberg Book Services,
166 East 56 Street, New York, New York 10022

ISBN: 0-440-20596-4

Printed in the United States of America
Published simultaneously in Canada

June 1990

10 9 8 7 6 5 4 3 2 1

OPM

# ACKNOWLEDGMENTS

The author would like to express her gratitude for the helpful suggestions contributed by Dr. Richard Wagman, Dr. Joyce Singer, Charles Berges, and Lynn Sonberg, and for the indispensable resources of the Arthritis Foundation.

# CONTENTS

# FOREWORD

Thirty-seven million Americans of all ages suffer from arthritis in one or another of its many forms. The disease occurs in one in every three families, and, because of its generally debilitating effect, arthritis tends to have an indirect impact on everyone in the family.

Arthritis is an umbrella term, covering more than 100 rheumatic diseases. Among the most prominent are osteoarthritis, or degenerative joint disease; rheumatoid arthritis, which, if uncontrolled, may destroy bone tissue; infectious arthritis; gout, brought on by a metabolic malfunction; and lupus, the most unpredictable form of arthritis. Lyme disease, communicated by ticks that live on deer and mice, and carpal tunnel syndrome, an inflammatory condition of the wrist, are also arthritis-like ailments.

Unfortunately, many inaccurate ideas about joint disease persist, as old wives' tales or folklore, and the result can be inadequate or wrongheaded attention to the very serious problems it brings. Often people who become involved with such beliefs and practices wait too long—in some cases, years—before consulting with a doctor about their symptoms. It is to be hoped that the information contained in this useful and authoritative book will motivate people to seek proper and timely treatment.

For the individual patient, correct diagnosis of the type of arthritis is of overwhelming importance. For example, patients with infectious arthritis must be treated with antibiotics, which are inappropriate for other types of the disease. Physicians should look into all possible medical causes, for a very large number exist. In addition, many factors in a patient's habits—at work and at leisure—may have given rise to arthritis.

Today's patients enjoy the benefits of many current advances in diagnostic technology. In addition to traditional blood and urine tests, X rays, and tissue examinations, doctors are now using many new technologies. Arthrocentesis, analysis of the fluid surrounding the joint, has improved diagnosis and treatment. CAT scan provides a three-dimensional image of the affected area. New techniques involving magnetism instead of X rays allow repeated examination without danger from radiation. Arthroscopy, illuminated visual examination through fiber optic technology, allows more precise examination and the performing of sophisticated therapeutic procedures.

Strictly construed, the goals of the treatment of arthritis are to provide the patient with relief from pain, to reduce and slow the process of inflammation, and to maintain a range of motion in the affected joints. Yet increasingly the definition of therapy has widened. Today physicians and other health professionals seek to enable people with arthritis to participate in their chosen activities and to live their lives to the fullest.

This expanded goal has given rise to the concept of a treatment team. Arthritis can have multiple causes, it often responds to treatment differently from patient to patient, and it affects many aspects of a person's life, depending on the degree of pain or immobility and the type of life the patient leads. Patients benefit from consulting not only with their primary physicians, but also with specialists in medication, protection devices and crutches, exercise and massage, corrective surgery, and other areas. Home aides, medical social workers, and psychologists can help sort out problems presented by the disease.

People with arthritis need not be relegated to lives of inactivity and constant pain. The key to finding the right team of professionals and the right treatment methods is to first acknowledge the very personal nature of this disease and thus the very personal nature of the treatment to be given. Patients must interact closely with their doctors in the search for the cause and best treatment.

To that end, this book serves as a valuable reference tool,

allowing patients to be knowledgeable as they seek to understand their illness. It provides a thorough discussion of medications, including questions to ask and caveats to bear in mind, as well as guidance for making a balanced assessment about the likely benefits of surgery. Importantly, it shows the reader how to participate in the design of an effective exercise regime.

The book is also to be recommended for its presentation of methods of practical self-help, including special devices for self-reliance, employment options, and support groups—especially important in a disease syndrome that, in addition to physical discomforts and incapacity, involves considerable uncertainty and unpredictability.

Medical researchers are learning much about the various forms of arthritis. They are learning more about the nature of inflammation and about the genetic aspects of the disease; research suggests that subtle defects in the immune system may allow arthritis to be more easily triggered. Other researchers are studying the ways joints fit together and move, and how they react to stress and strain, in an effort to develop better strengthening exercises and advice on postures, as well as equipment that will prevent damage to bones and tissues.

Meanwhile, *Relief from Chronic Arthritis Pain* is a valuable sourcebook of the best current information, pointing arthritis sufferers and family members in many directions for meaningful help. Most significantly, it allows the patient to become an active partner with the doctor or treatment team in determining medications and practices that allow a mode of living that is fuller and more comfortable than was thought possible even a few years ago.

RICHARD WAGMAN, M.D.
*Associate Professor of Clinical Medicine*
*State University of New York*
*Health Science Center at Brooklyn*

# ONE

# KNOWING THE
# FACTS CAN HELP
# YOU COPE

"Take lots of vitamin E." ... "Don't ever eat eggplant." ...
"Mudbaths are like magic." ... "Aspirin is still the best
medicine." ... "Stay away from *all* medicine and take an
herbal mixture."

There's no shortage of advice out there about arthritis.
Unfortunately, much of it isn't helpful, and some of it can be
harmful. Part of the problem is that the term *arthritis* is a
catchall for about a hundred different conditions, and the
symptoms of many of them seem to come and go for no
apparent reason.

The Arthritis Foundation estimates that of the 37 million
Americans trying to cope with one or another form of arthritis, a significant number need competent medical treatment
and aren't getting it. Some of these sufferers accept their
misery as an inevitable aspect of aging. Others, who refuse to
have anything to do with established treatments, waste time
and money on fraudulent "cures."

While it's true that most forms of arthritis can't be cured,
they can all be treated. There are effective ways of relieving
pain, both medically and nonmedically. Many different drugs
are available for successfully fighting the damage resulting
from inflammation. Crippling can be avoided, or if it has
occurred already, it can be reduced or even overcome by

1

innovative surgery. Patients and their families can receive professional guidance in the methods for preserving normal joint function. Family counselors, psychotherapists, and support groups can be called on to help preserve social relationships and job responsibilities.

## SOME COMMON MISCONCEPTIONS

*"I'm too young to have arthritis."* Joint disease can occur at any age, including childhood. A teenager can suffer from chronically painful joints because of inadequately treated Lyme disease. A young woman may develop a troublesome case of infectious arthritis secondary to a gonorrhea infection. Rheumatoid arthritis may suddenly attack a man who is otherwise healthy and in the prime of life.

*"Doctors don't know the cause and they don't have a cure, so why should I waste my money on diagnostic tests?"* One of the main purposes of this book is to spell out the various ways in which the many forms of arthritis *can be treated.* In most cases the crippling effects are *not* inevitable if the right steps are taken early enough. There are new medicines and many ways of controlling pain; progressive joint damage can be slowed down and even halted with the combined participation of the patient, physician, physical therapist, and family members.

*"If I watch what I eat and go to yoga classes, my aches and pains will disappear."* Degenerative joint disease or inflammation isn't the result of what you eat and drink (except in some cases of gout). Yoga classes may be relaxing, but there are specific exercises designed to maintain the range of motion of arthritic joints if they're done regularly.

*"When I feel stiff and achy, I take a drink or a tranquilizer, and I feel better right away."* Getting hooked on alcohol and/or pills to get through the day or to fall asleep is a dangerous way to deal with arthritis—or any other ailment. The fact that you feel more "relaxed" doesn't mean that the joint damage isn't progressing, perhaps to a point where no amount of later correct treatment can undo the harm.

## WHERE DOES ARTHRITIS HAPPEN?

The term *arthritis* literally means *inflammation of a joint.* Some forms cause only minor discomfort and don't interfere with normal functioning; others can disrupt every aspect of one's life, and almost all forms are chronic. Nearly all of us, men and women alike, will have to deal with some form of rheumatic ailment as we move beyond our sixtieth birthdays. It's therefore helpful to know that whether your painful joint is located in your fingers or your feet, your knee or your hip, a joint is structurally the same everywhere in your body. It is the place where two bones join together and are surrounded by the components illustrated below.

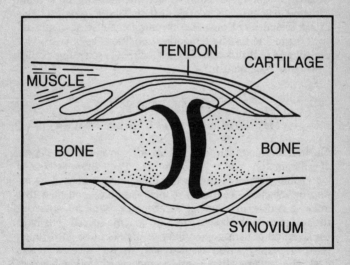

The cartilage that covers the ends of the bones is a tissue strong enough to take lots of wear, elastic enough to act as a shock absorber, and as slippery as ice to keep the bones from rubbing against each other. The joint is surrounded by a sac called the *synovium,* whose lining, the synovial membrane, secretes a lubricating fluid. The synovial fluid enters the narrow space between the bones, and at the same time that it nourishes the cartilage, it also contributes to the smooth functioning of the joint. Ligaments, tendons, and muscles are the connective tissue that give strength and support to the bones during the performance of their many movements. Ligaments are tough, fibrous cords that connect the bones to each other. Tendons are similarly tough bands that connect muscle and bone. Scattered through the connective tissues are pouches called *bursae*—the Latin for purses or bags—containing a small amount of fluid. They are usually located in fibrous tissue at a point where there is likely to be constant pressure or friction.

The various kinds of arthritis that affect the normal functioning of the joints come under the heading of a more inclusive group of disorders called *rheumatic diseases*. This group includes not only the chronic joint diseases, but also such acute and usually temporary conditions as bursitis, tendinitis, and fibrositis. This latter condition is sometimes called "muscular rheumatism."

## INFLAMMATION: THE WARNING THAT GOES AWRY

All the more common forms of arthritis involve some degree of inflammation *within the joint*. The inflammation associated with joint diseases is unlike the inflammation caused by injury or infection. The heat, redness, swelling, and pain that follow a bruise, or a cut, or a bacterial or viral infection are the response of the body's immune system. Special cells heed the warning of damage by injury or invasion and go through the processes of defense and repair. As the affected tissues heal, the inflammation subsides and vanishes. We have all lived through such episodes of inflammation followed by total recovery: a tender puffy gum around an infected tooth; a hot, painfully swollen knee following a fall; a "sore" throat.

In many types of arthritis, however, the inflammation is no mere warning. It becomes the problem in itself, attacking healthy tissues, wearing them down, and damaging cartilage and bones to the point where they become misshapen. This process of self-perpetuating inflammation can be extremely painful and eventually disabling if it isn't controlled by suitable treatment.

## WHEN YOU SHOULD CONSULT A DOCTOR

Be alert to the message your body is sending. The right treatment at the right time can spare you lots of misery. Make an appointment with your doctor if you experience any of the following symptoms over a period of several weeks:

- persistent stiffness accompanied by some pain when you get up in the morning.

- pain, redness, swelling, or tenderness to the touch in one or more joints.

- joint-pains that interfere with sleep during the night.

- increasing clumsiness or difficulty in doing normal tasks on the job and at home.

- numbness or tingling sensations in fingers and toes.

- persistent pain in the hips, knees, or neck.

- fatigue or weakness, fever, and unexplained weight loss combined with aching joints.

## WHY DIAGNOSIS IS IMPORTANT

Because there are many different kinds of arthritis, a precise diagnosis is essential before the correct treatment can begin. Accuracy takes time. Your cooperation is essential in giving a detailed medical history that includes family illnesses as well as your own. Blood tests, urine analysis, tissue biopsies, tests of the synovial fluids, and X rays may be necessary in order to distinguish one type of arthritis from another, and making this distinction is essential before the right treatment can begin. If, for example, you have infectious arthritis brought on by a bacterial disease, you'll need a course of the right antibiotics as soon as possible to knock out the basic cause. But antibiotics don't do any good at all if your joint inflammation is a symptom of rheumatoid arthritis. And if it turns out that your aches and pains can be attributed to degenerative joint disease—the wear and tear from arthritis common to the elderly—you may be advised to take aspirin on a regular basis, even when you're no longer distressed by pain and stiffness.

## BUILDING A WORKING RELATIONSHIP WITH THE RIGHT DOCTOR

Since you're likely to be in for the long haul when you have arthritis, try to find a doctor who you feel is patient and understanding, who answers your questions, and who takes the time to listen to you. The most effective doctors are, and have always been, those who see their patients not as a bundle of symptoms but as whole human beings; who treat the individual person and not the disease. Holistic health care in the most desirable sense is not some offbeat unconventional approach to "healing." Many conventional physicians make a point of asking patients not only the standard questions about past illnesses. They also want to know about your interpersonal relationships and stresses within the family; what kind of work you do and how you feel about it, as well as whether the work is sedentary or involves movement; how you spend your leisure time; whether you exercise regularly; what a typical day's meals might consist of; how your vacations are spent and with whom; how much alcohol you consume, and what other drugs—legal and illegal, prescription and nonprescription—you take regularly. A good doctor who makes an effort to create an atmosphere of mutual respect won't call you by your first name at the same time that you're expected to use a formal "Dr. So-and-So" in return.

Doctors who can be trusted know the limitations of their

expertise. If, for example, your doctor wants a confirmation of the diagnosis of rheumatoid arthritis or systemic lupus erythematosus, you may be referred to a rheumatologist. Another possibility is team treatment at an outpatient clinic where health professionals from a variety of specialties will be available to treat all of your problems in one location. (For more information on rheumatology and team treatment, see Chapter Eight, pages 87–88).

## PATIENT PARTICIPATION: THE KEY TO SUCCESSFUL MANAGEMENT

Whatever form of arthritis you're coping with, the basic goals of treatment are the same: relief of pain, reduction of inflammation, and the maintenance—if possible, the improvement—of the range of motion of the affected joints.

Unlike other chronic conditions in which patient participation consists mainly in taking a particular medicine or losing weight or avoiding certain foods, successful arthritis treatment demands your understanding and active involvement at every step of the treatment. In order to create a program that suits your particular needs, you and your physician have to work out the right combination of medicine; special exercises; a balance of rest, relaxation, and participation in normal activities, and joint protection when necessary. You may also be expected to change old posture habits, and you may be advised to give serious consideration to changing your job if your condition appears to be occupation-related.

## GUIDELINES AND SUGGESTIONS

Oftentimes doctors and other health professionals may be too busy to answer your questions. The purpose of the pages that follow is to anticipate many of these questions and provide you and your family with helpful information: how to recognize the symptoms of the more common forms of arthritis; how they are diagnosed and treated medically and surgically;

the role of the physical therapist and how you can be helped in achieving a good balance of exercise and rest; where to find the latest useful objects especially designed to simplify your daily life if you're somewhat disabled; what options you have for getting relief from pain if you've tried the anti-inflammatory medications and they don't work for you; how to evaluate the role of special diets, megavitamins, chiropractic, homeopathy, and other conventional treatments, and how you can recognize quackery so that you're not seduced into squandering your money on false cures.

# TWO

# DEGENERATIVE JOINT DISEASE (Osteoarthritis): Usually Age-Related and Usually Benign

In the beginning you might notice stiff creaky joints that feel fine after a hot shower, but within a few months your hip really hurts. Or you might notice that your knee seems to be giving you trouble ever since that bad fall. And what are those funny red bumps that have begun to appear on your finger joints? In all likelihood you're developing the most common form of arthritis—degenerative joint disease.

This chapter will give you an understanding of what happens in your body to cause episodes of stiffness and pain, how the condition can worsen if ignored, and the advances in technology that make an accurate diagnosis possible if any doubts exist about the nature of your ailment. One of the most exciting of these advances has occurred in a field called *arthroscopy*, which is described in some detail on page 20.

In addition to a summary of treatments, you'll also find some helpful suggestions for self-management. Many additional suggestions are contained in the chapters on medicine, surgery, exercise, and pain control, especially in the chapter on helping yourself and getting help from others.

# A CLOSER LOOK AT
# TERMINOLOGY

The term *osteoarthritis* was introduced into the medical lexicon more than a hundred years ago, and from that time to this specialists have been trying to redefine and refine the standards for this disease category. Some of us are old enough to remember venerable family members who talked about their "rheumatism" when they complained about an aching hip or bumpy finger joints. According to the American Rheumatology Association and to the specialists known since 1940 as "rheumatologists," what they were probably talking about is now professionally known as *degenerative joint disease,* the most common of all the arthritic disorders. It is the disorder characterized by slowly developing joint stiffness and pain, some joint enlargement, and some limitation of movement. It is associated with aging, during which there is a gradual deterioration of the cartilage between the bone surfaces of the joints.

The designation *primary osteoarthritis* is now increasingly reserved for the less common inflammatory condition that is characterized by greater pain, redness, swelling, and deformity than its degenerative counterpart. However, keep in mind that final distinctions have not yet been conclusively made, and that there is sometimes an overlapping between the degenerative and inflammatory aspects. The critical distinction is the placing of these two disorders in one category so that they can be distinguished from *rheumatoid arthritis,* which is discussed in the next chapter.

# A CLOSER LOOK AT
# THE AILMENT

The main defect in cases of degenerative joint disease is cartilage deterioration, most commonly in the joints of the fingers, knees, hips, and, when the spine is involved, in the cervical vertebrae (the neck). The weight-bearing joints—knees and hips—are especially vulnerable. Only in rare cases is the elbow affected, and ankle involvement is likely to be related to your occupation rather than to your age.

As the cartilage begins to deteriorate its surface becomes roughened. And as the process continues the articulating ends of the bones that form the joints are increasingly deprived of the smooth protective layer of cartilage that enables them to slide smoothly over each other. In parts of the bone where cartilage deterioration is most advanced, cyst-like formations may occur. Cases monitored by X rays show that these cysts are most likely to appear in the hip. When the cysts collapse the result is likely to be deformity of the bone. The ongoing deterioration of cartilage also leads to the formation of bony projections called *spurs* at the margins of the affected joints. When spurs form the joint space narrows, further interfering with smooth function.

## CARTILAGE—THE CRITICAL COMPONENT

Anyone who has ever cut up a raw chicken or has been able to wheedle soup bones from a butcher knows that the ends of bones are covered with a shiny, blue-white, very slippery surface. This covering is cartilage, a special type of supporting tissue that, together with bone, makes up the skeleton. In its earliest stage the entire skeleton is made up of cartilage, and as the process of bone formation occurs in the fetus, cartilage remains only at the ends of the bones, where it serves as the articular surface of the joints.

In the broadest sense degenerative joint disease begins when there is a defect in the cartilage such that cartilage repair does not keep pace with cartilage erosion.

## CAUSES OF CARTILAGE EROSION

There is an ever-greater understanding of the underlying reasons for the degeneration of one of the body's toughest tissues. The old explanation that was supposed to cover all cases of creaking and painful joints—"It's an inevitable part of aging"—is no longer considered universally applicable. After all, there are many people in their seventies and eighties whose X rays may show tissue deterioration, but you'd never know—and they don't seem to show—that they have a disability of any kind. On the other hand, there are some men and women in their forties and fifties who have a hard time getting out of bed in the morning because of a stiff and painful hip or knee.

It is generally agreed that many factors—genetic, metabolic, biochemical, and structural—can play a critical role in cartilage degeneration. Here are some causes that might apply in your case:

• Is one of your legs shorter than the other or have you had a dislocated hip since birth?

• Have you had any injuries to your knee or thigh joint that weren't properly treated?

• Over the years have you engaged in active sports without regard to possible joint overuse? Do you constantly play squash or tennis or participate in bicycle races?

• Do you have the kind of job that involves day-in, day-out overuse of particular joints comparable to bus driver's shoulders, ballet dancer's hips, or violinist's wrists?

• Are the joints of your right hand deteriorating because you're exclusively right-handed in all your manual labor?

Other factors about which patients are unaware until they are revealed by detailed laboratory tests include:

• The release of body substances that cause the deterioration of collagen, one of the structural parts of cartilage. There is very little information about what triggers the release of these destructive substances.

• Minor fractures that occur with less than normal impact because of the deteriorated collagen, thereby speeding up the wearing away of the cartilage.

• Inflammation resulting from an accumulation of crystal deposits on the inside or outside of joint cartilage.

## EARLY WARNING SIGNALS

Degenerative joint disease doesn't begin dramatically. You're not going to have an acute attack of pain or fever that would send you to the doctor for immediate treatment. This form of arthritis begins slowly and gradually. The discomfort is local rather than generalized. There comes a time when your hip or knee might feel painful after a long walk, and a nagging soreness might persist for about fifteen minutes. In these early stages you can get rid of the discomfort by resting with your feet up or relaxing in a warm bath.

Another warning to watch for is a feeling of creakiness in joints that are required to move after you've been sitting in the same position for a long time. This sensation of stiffness when you wake up in the morning is probably the most common complaint of older people. It is usually the first sign that cartilage deterioration has begun.

## HOW DEGENERATIVE JOINT
## DISEASE PROGRESSES

Maybe you can control these minor aches and pains on your own with the help of aspirin and periods of rest. But in many cases, when the first signals are ignored or it's assumed that nothing can be done about them, the condition gradually worsens. At this stage pain is experienced in the affected joint with the slightest movement. Sometimes the pain might be sharp enough to interrupt sleep. (The pain arises from structures in and around the joint and not from the eroded cartilage, since cartilage, having no nerve supply, is entirely insensitive.) As the degeneration continues, the cartilage becomes pitted and increasingly eroded to the point where the surface of the bone itself is exposed. Following this exposure, spurs and cysts form on the bone, and the bone surface below the eroding cartilage becomes thicker and harder. If inflammation of the synovial membrane (synovitis) occurs because of crystal deposits or because of advanced degeneration of surrounding tissues, the area becomes painful not only at the slightest movement but also at the lightest touch.

At this advanced stage the joint is likely to become enlarged and somewhat misshapen.

## SOME SPECIFICS ABOUT AFFECTED AREAS

### Hands

While you're filing your nails you might suddenly become aware of a small sore bump on the top joint of the right-hand index finger. When you examine your left hand you notice that a similar bony red bump is beginning to develop in exactly the same place on the left index finger. It's not unusual for these bony spurs on the top joints to develop symmetrically. They are called *Heberden's nodes,* memorializing the eighteenth-century English doctor who first observed them as a characteristic of "the rheumatism," especially in women.

They may begin right after an injury or trauma to the hand, or they may develop for no apparent reason. To start with they are likely to be painful, itchy, and red, but in time the soreness goes and only the hard bump remains. They're scarcely noticeable by anyone but the person who has them, and they don't interfere in any way with normal finger function.

Degenerative joint disease in the fingers that begins with stiffness and some pain should be attended to promptly so that irreversible deformities don't occur. Some older people do have gnarled hands that have no impairment of function, but it's a good idea to prevent misshapen joints by consulting your doctor as soon as they begin to feel stiff and sore. (Increasing pain and immobility may indicate the presence of carpal tunnel syndrome, discussed in Chapter Four.)

**HELPFUL HINTS:** Stiffness in the fingers is almost always eased by daily exercise. (See illustration, page 77 for illustrated suggestion.) It can also be reduced by wearing nylon spandex stretch gloves, especially during sleep. The warmth provided by these gloves throughout the night makes the fingers more flexible and more limber than they would otherwise be in the morning. A finger joint that has suddenly become inflamed should be immobilized by a splint. After a period of enforced rest, and a suitable dosage of aspirin or some other anti-inflammatory drug, it will recover. The splinting is just as important as the medication. If you think the pains in your fingers are caused by overuse in a hobby (needlepoint is a common culprit) or by occupational demands, monitor your leisure activities more closely; if necessary, see if you can arrange a temporary job change. And among the easiest and oldest ways to reduce pain is the application of heat—either by soaking in warm water or covering the sore areas with warm paraffin wax.

## Knee

Most of us have childhood memories of scraped knees, bruised knees, even a dislocated knee as the result of a fall. Kneecap injuries are a common occurrence in adulthood too. If you participate in racket sports, or you're a daily runner or bicycle rider, you've probably had your share of such injuries, a consequence of which may be a condition called *chondromalacia patellae*. In this condition the cartilage that cushions the undersurface of the kneecap becomes increasingly soft. It is a form of degenerative joint disease likely to affect young adults who regularly indulge in active sports.

Deterioration of knee cartilage in older people is common among those who are overweight or whose lifetime of poor posture has caused the knee joint to move out of its normal position.

A painful knee can be very painful indeed, and the pain is intensified when walking up and down stairs or walking on hilly ground. It can also be dangerous if the knee joint "locks" and causes the knee to buckle. If this happens when stepping down from a curb or walking downstairs, the result may be a serious accident involving a hip injury.

Any suspicion of knee problems should therefore be investigated by your doctor without delay.

HELPFUL HINTS: If for any reason your knee begins to feel sore or you're unsteady on your feet from time to time because the joint feels wobbly, ask the doctor whether an elastic support of the kneecap will give the joint the necessary stability. Find out whether it would be worthwhile to undergo surgery for realigning the joint so that healthy cartilage surfaces can be brought into the correct position. Knee problems mean that you have to give up jogging, perhaps permanently. If being overweight is contributing to the problem, don't do any crash dieting. Join Weight Watchers or ask your doctor to help you work out a weight-loss program that you'll be able to maintain indefinitely. (Some people find it helpful to join a support group like Overeaters Anonymous while their weight is stabilizing.) Jogging will have to be given up in favor of some other form of regular exercise (swimming is a good substitute). If poor posture is part of the knee problem, discuss a practical solution with your doctor, such as a referral to a physical therapist. Above all, don't participate in any exercise programs involving the knee without the doctor's permission.

## Hip

There's no explanation for the fact that the degeneration of a hip joint may look quite extensive on an X ray, and yet many years may pass before any troublesome symptoms appear. It's also not unusual for hip pain to come and go, sometimes disappearing altogether for months at a time. When the pain is present it's usually localized in the groin, and it may also travel along the inner surface of the thigh. Because certain nerve paths are close together, pain originating in the hip may transfer to the buttocks by way of the sciatic nerve.

Sometimes the pain may be intense or frequent enough to cause a limp.

HELPFUL HINTS: Degenerative joint disease of the hip should be treated as soon as painful twinges begin so that tissue damage is kept to a minimum. Eventual immobilization can be prevented in most cases with a regular program of heat and rest combined with the right amount of an anti-inflammatory drug. If obesity is a contributing factor, weight loss should be part of the treatment program. If posture needs correcting, attention should be given to exercises that will lead to improvement. If necessary, a cane should be used to reduce the weight-bearing stress on the hip; in more severe cases a walker should be considered. However, the recent advances in hip surgery, and especially in hip replacement, have enabled many people well along in years to abandon their wheelchairs. (Surgical options are discussed in detail in Chapter Six.)

## Spine

Cartilage degeneration in the vertebrae can proceed to the point where spurs begin to appear on the bone. When they do appear they cause the narrowing of the opening through which the nerves must pass. This combined circumstance—the development of the spurs and the narrowing of the space—causes the spurs to press on the nerve. When this happens the pain can be severe enough to be immobilizing, and it can become even more intense because when the nerve is irritated it swells, thereby increasing the pressure it is subjected to.

When bony spurs develop under the cartilage in the vertebrae of the lower spine, pressure is placed on one or the other sciatic nerve and the result is similar to sciatica. Because the sciatic nerves are the longest in the body, extending from the lower spine through the buttocks, thighs, and calves down to the lower leg, irritation of one or both of the nerves, from no matter what source, can produce twinges of pain along its entire path.

HELPFUL HINTS: Getting an accurate diagnosis may take time, but it's time well spent. Back pain is a problem shared by millions of men and women, but the source can be attributed to a wide range of conditions, each with its own treatment. Tests and X rays may indicate that you don't have arthritis at all, that what you need is a chair with a good back support or a weight-loss and exercise program. When it turns out that degenerative joint disease *is* the cause, you and your doctor can work out a schedule of rest and medication that will control the pain and keep inflammation at a minimum. Severe pain in the lower spine can also be relieved by a corset designed to provide abdominal support. When painkilling drugs don't entirely ease the discomfort in the area of the neck, a cervical collar can be helpful. (Other options for pain management are discussed in Chapters Eight and Nine.)

## CLOSING IN ON THE
## RIGHT DIAGNOSIS

It wasn't too long ago that older patients who complained to the doctor about aching joints were told to go home, use a heating pad, lie down from time to time, and take two aspirins. If the complaints continued, further investigation would involve X rays to determine the extent of the joint damage and, where it seemed advisable, surgery might have been recommended. Nowadays, however, a conscientious doctor confronted with complaints about aching joints with symptoms of inflammation uses recently developed diagnostic tools to make the correct diagnosis.

Before deciding that the problem is indeed degenerative joint disease, various tests are given to rule out the possibility of rheumatoid arthritis. (These tests are described in the next chapter.) A detailed history and blood tests also determine whether the inflammation comes under the heading of infectious arthritis secondary to a bacterial infection such as gonorrhea or Lyme disease.

Another ambiguity has to be resolved: Is the onset of pain

in the knee or hip caused not by cartilage deterioration as such but by crystal deposits under the cartilage or in the synovial fluid?

# ADVANCES IN MEDICAL TECHNOLOGY

There have been many advances in medical practice that affect diagnostic accuracy. Most doctors now take greater care in writing up a patient's medical history, asking for information not only about illnesses, surgery, and the like but also about family disease patterns, the precise nature of one's job, leisure activities, and so on. But it is the advances in medical technology dating from the 1950s that enable a well-informed and well-equipped prime-care doctor—and certainly a rheumatologist—to arrive at a more refined diagnosis than ever before, thus making more effective treatment possible.

The use of *computerized axial tomography*, otherwise known as a CAT scan, is especially effective in clarifying conditions beyond the scope of traditional X ray. This is accomplished by using radiography to construct a three-dimensional picture of a body structure so that the various layers of tissue are visible. With this diagnostic tool your doctor can find out whether the persistent pain in your spine is caused by a herniated disc or cartilage degeneration. A CAT scan can also differentiate between a primary neurological disorder and a neurological abnormality caused by degenerative joint disease.

*Magnetic resonance imaging* (MRI) is a noninvasive diagnostic tool that uses magnetism instead of X rays to provide visual information. Because it offers sharp, clear contrasts, it is especially suitable for imaging the musculoskeletal system, whose components have an unusually broad range of tissue densities. Thus if a doctor feels that X rays of your painful knee don't provide enough detailed visual information about possible tiny lesions or cysts, this type of imaging will be used. It has the additional advantage that it can be used over and over again to track the effectiveness of a cure, since, unlike X rays, it doesn't subject the patient to the potentially damaging effects of overexposure to radiation.

## ARTHROSCOPY

The advancing technology of fiber optics has led to the creation of many instruments such as the arthroscope that enable the physician to throw a sharply focused light on internal parts of your body previously inaccessible to inspection. Because it can illuminate parts of the joint previously inaccessible to other instruments except in surgical procedures, the arthroscope has proved particularly helpful in diagnosing osteoarthritic problems. In the past two decades arthroscopy has become indispensable in surgery as well.

For example, minor surgical procedures used early in the course of degenerative joint disease or inflammatory osteoarthritis have halted tissue destruction and reduced pain to a minimum. Through arthroscopy a diseased joint can be irrigated and healthy tissue can be exposed by the removal of devitalized debris. Irrigation can also remove fragments of deteriorated cartilage from synovial fluid.

Another procedure made possible by arthroscopy is the use of abrasion to remove degenerated cartilage almost down to the bone in the hope that healthy functional cartilage will be regenerated.

## ARTHROCENTESIS:
## "LIQUID BIOPSY OF A JOINT"

Just as amniocentesis is proving invaluable in providing obstetricians and parents-to-be with critical information about fetal development, arthrocentesis is providing essential information for rheumatologists and their patients. The technique in both cases consists of withdrawing a sample of fluid through a hollow needle that has been inserted into the designated area.

If, for instance, your doctor wants to find out whether you have infectious osteoarthritis or crystal-induced osteoarthritis, using arthrocentesis to analyze the synovial fluid is considered by specialists to be the only reliable way to make the differentiation. If your joint inflammation is caused by bacterial infection, the count of white blood cells in the synovial fluid will be higher than normal. Such a finding hastens correct treatment—in this case antibiotics to knock out the infection, thereby preventing further tissue inflammation.

## TIME FOR TREATMENT

When a battery of tests indicates that you have osteoarthritis or degenerative joint disease rather than any other form of arthritis, treatment will be individualized to suit *your* body, *your* reactions to various medications, and *your* way of life.

You can learn more about these choices in Chapters Five through Nine. Whatever treatment program you embark on, stay with it, consult regularly with your doctor, and don't be discouraged if it takes time and effort to get good results. More help is out there than ever before. Knowing how to use it is one of the best guarantees of successful treatment.

# THREE

# RHEUMATOID ARTHRITIS:
## Prompt Treatment Means Better Management

There was a time—and it wasn't too long ago—when the recommended treatment for people with rheumatoid arthritis was total rest—which meant living out one's allotted years as a bedridden invalid. Fortunately, for the millions of Americans who have this disease,* such is no longer the case. While it remains one of the more disabling forms of arthritis, it has become much easier to manage, thanks to more effective medicines, advances in surgery, a better understanding of how pain can be controlled, and a wide range of supports, both physical and psychological. One of the most profound differences is this: If you have rheumatoid arthritis, you need no longer be a passive victim. With team guidance you can take charge of many aspects of your treatment and lead an active, productive life. Your prime-care physician may refer you to a rheumatologist who will help you find the medication that produces the best results for *you.* Together with the physical therapist, you can develop an exercise and rest routine suitable for the demands of your daily life. An orthopedic surgeon can spell out various options that will increase your

---

*The Arthritis Foundation estimates that about 1 percent of the adult population in the United States has rheumatoid arthritis, or about 2.5 million people. Of this number, three quarters are women.

mobility and reduce your pain, and the team's social worker can instruct family members in differentiating between those situations when you need to be helped and those when your efforts to be independent should be supported.

A great deal of mystery and misunderstanding continue to surround rheumatoid arthritis. The information that follows in this chapter and others should enable patients and their families to cope more effectively with this disease. It should also enable others to be alert to its symptoms.

## WHAT IS RHEUMATOID ARTHRITIS?

Rheumatoid arthritis is a chronic disease characterized by on-and-off inflammation of the joints. If the inflammation continues uncontrolled, the result may be irreversible destruction of bone tissue. It is usually described as a systemic disease because it affects the functioning of the entire body. It used to be thought that involvement of the heart or lungs or blood vessels was a secondary complication of the joint inflammation, but these involvements are now seen as part of the disease itself.

If you've had a siege of the flu, you've experienced achy feelings in your knees and your neck that keep you in bed for a few days, but eventually the aches in your joints go away and you're fine again. With the onset of rheumatoid arthritis the symptoms don't go away. They persist, and if not treated properly, they get worse. The early signs are:

- swelling, redness, and soreness in any joint—hips, knees, ankles, toes, wrists, fingers, neck—and usually in the corresponding joint on the other side of the body;

- persistent warmth and tenderness to the touch of any joint;

- severe pain that prevents normal movement of any joint;

- in combination with joint-pain, fever, and feelings of fatigue that come and go and weight loss unconnected with changes in eating habits.

## WHY DO SOME PEOPLE
## GET RHEUMATOID ARTHRITIS
## AND OTHERS DON'T?

There are many theories about the cause of rheumatoid arthritis, and research scientists are investigating all of them so that eventually it will be possible to find a cure or, better still, to prevent its occurrence. Exhaustive studies show that where you live, how you earn your living, what you eat, and your personality type may affect the *course* of the disease, but none of these factors have so far been proved to be part of the cause. Some researchers believe a virus is responsible; others are exploring the mysteries of the immune system. In the meantime it has become clear that several factors do *predispose* some people to the disease:

### Genetic tendency

There is now compelling evidence that some people have inherited a tendency toward rheumatoid arthritis. This supposition is supported by the fact that the majority of people with RA have the same specific genetic marker or tissue type, called *HLA-DR4*. (A tissue type is similar to a blood type.) However, having HLA-DR4 tissue type does not mean you will develop RA. HLA-DR4 is a common tissue type shared by about 25 percent of the population, most of whom will never get rheumatoid arthritis. What "genetic tendency" means is that those who belong to this tissue type are at greater risk for developing the disease.

### Rheumatoid factor

About 80 percent of RA patients have an abnormal antibody in their blood and joint fluid. This rheumatoid factor is a protein that interacts with the immune system in such a way that the body essentially becomes allergic to itself. Whatever the triggering mechanism might be, the inflammation process becomes cumulative. It doesn't subside as it normally would once a virus is overcome or injured tissue has healed. In RA the inflammation itself stimulates the release of destructive substances that result in more damage to joint tissue, leading to more inflammation. Thus a primary purpose of treatment is to interrupt and control what appears to be a chain reaction.

## RESULTS OF DELAYED TREATMENT

If rheumatoid arthritis isn't treated promptly, it can lead to loss of joint function in a series of irreversible steps. (See illustration.)

(1) Inflammation begins in the synovial membrane that lines the capsule containing the joint. The rheumatoid factor—or some as yet unknown factor—triggers the synovial cells into sending an antibody into the joint space, thereby initiating the disease process.

(2) As the inflammation takes hold the synovial membrane begins to manufacture a new tissue called *pannus,* which grows like a tumor and begins to erode the joint cartilage.

(3) In the process of growth the pannus formation irreversibly damages cartilage, tendons, and bone surface.

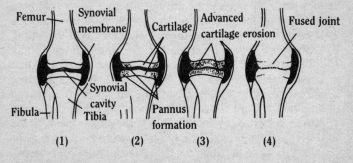

(4) The joint cavity is totally destroyed, and the bones forming the joint—in this case the knee—are fused together. When this fusion occurs inflammation stops, pain is at an end, and joint mobility is lost.

## UNPREDICTABILITY IS PART OF THE PATTERN

One of the most mystifying aspects of the RA process is the fact that the symptoms vary not only from person to person but for the same person on different days. Following a period of severe inflammation, during which swelling, redness, and pain of the fingers or the ankles make movement practically impossible, the symptoms will diminish, or they might even disappear altogether. There seems to be no way of accounting for these periods of remission, which might last for days or weeks, or even for years. In fact, for about 20 percent of all cases, especially for those people who have had the disease for only a year or so, all the symptoms disappear forever, even though laboratory findings show that it is still present. For others, however, the periods of remission are inevitably followed by flares or flare-ups. At these times the symptoms may become more acute than they were previously.

Sometimes flares follow a stressful situation, such as a quarrel or a visit from a divorced child with lots of problems; sometimes they might be attributable to a nasty cold or a sudden drop in temperature. In general, since there appears to be no way of predicting them, there's no way of preventing them. But there *are* effective ways of coping with them.

Unfortunately, it's the very fact of unpredictability that causes many people to delay diagnosis, falsely assuming that the periods of remission mean that their problems aren't too serious. There are also those people who try this or that quack "cure," convinced by charlatans that the snake venom or the copper bracelet caused their symptoms to go away. They go to spas, they go to nutritionists, they go to all types of "healers." In fact, they go to everyone but a competent doctor. According to the Arthritis Foundation, people wait, on the average, four years after the onset of symptoms before they make an effort to get a medical opinion. And in the meantime preventable progressive damage to the affected joints is taking place.

## A FIRM DIAGNOSIS
## TAKES TIME

Say that you are someone who doesn't ignore the signals your body sends you. A few years ago, when you were increasingly troubled by shortness of breath and wheezing, you didn't simply decide to "take it easy" when walking up and down stairs, you wanted to know whether it was your heart or the sudden onset of asthma or some other problem that needed taking care of. You made an appointment for a checkup, a diagnosis, and suitable treatment. The problem turned out to be asthma.

Now you wake up several mornings in succession with unaccustomed stiffness in the finger joints of both hands. In a few weeks the joints become red, swollen, and painful. You notice that your knees are beginning to get red and painful too. This doesn't seem like the aches and pains your mother has been coping with; her joints aren't red and tender to the touch. Off you go to the doctor.

Your medical records, your family history are taken out of the files and closely checked. New questions are asked about recent infections, recent emotional disturbances, new symptoms. Have you been losing weight? Do you feel more fatigued than usual? A complete physical examination follows. The affected joints are carefully scrutinized and gently squeezed to see how tender they are to the touch. (They *hurt*.) You get more and more anxious and want to know if you're going to end up in a wheelchair. The doctor is reassuring; there's no pooh-poohing response to your anxiety, but there's no quick diagnosis either. This will not be forthcoming until the results of several laboratory findings are evaluated. Among these are blood tests—one for the rheumatoid factor, another for the sedimentation rate. (This test measures the rate at which red blood cells drop to the bottom of a glass tube. If chronic inflammation is present, the cells fall more quickly than would normally occur.) A blood test may be done in the doctor's office to find out if you're anemic. A urine sample is also examined.

One of the most important tests involves the withdrawal of synovial fluid from one of the affected joints to find out whether infectious agents are the possible cause of the inflammation. Although X rays may be taken, they don't necessarily show any damage to the joints early in the course of rheumatoid arthritis. (X rays will probably be taken from time to time in the future to check on the effectiveness of treatment in controlling the course of tissue destruction.)

It may not be until your second or third visit and some follow-up tests that a diagnosis of rheumatoid arthritis will be confirmed.

## THE TREATMENT PROGRAM

Every treatment program for rheumatoid arthritis is tailored to fit the individual needs and circumstances of the patient. The goal at every stage is to control the inflammation, thereby keeping joint destruction at a minimum; to reduce the pain to the point where it doesn't interfere with normal activities; to keep you functioning at maximum capability in your community, during your leisure pursuits, in friendships, and in social activities. Various specialists who make up the treatment team may be consulted from time to time: a rheumatologist to make recommendations about a new medication; a physiatrist to make evaluations for joint-protection devices, crutches, or a special exercise program; a physical therapist, who may use massage or exercises involving weights during office visits and who visits you at home during periods of flare that keep you housebound but able to continue some exercises with help; an orthopedic surgeon, who may recommend that you consider joint realignment or joint replacement.

If you're being treated at a hospital outpatient rheumatology clinic, other staff members may be consulted as well: a social worker to help you resolve problems relating to your job or your need for a homemaking aide when you can't manage on your own; a psychiatrist or psychologist, who can offer essential counseling about dealing with stress and episodes of depression.

These and other aspects of treatment, including ingenious ways of helping yourself, unconventional healing approaches, and pain control are discussed in detail beginning on page 136.

If you're one of the two and a half million people coping with rheumatoid arthritis, try to keep in mind that no matter how bad the situation may seem, there *are* ways of making it better. Your treatment team can help you only up to a point; patience, determination, and a willingness to explore routes to pain relief are up to you.

# ARTHRITIS-RELATED DISORDERS:
## Infectious Arthritis, Gout, Systemic Lupus Erythematosus, Lyme Disease, and Carpal Tunnel Syndrome

The disorders discussed in the pages that follow differ significantly in cause and treatment, but they are all characterized by some degree of joint involvement. Infectious arthritis, for example, has many underlying causes, and treatment must begin with a secure diagnosis if it is to be at all effective. Gout is unlike most other types of arthritis because its cause is known to be a metabolic fault that can be corrected and controlled by specific medications unrelated to anti-inflammatory drugs. Systemic lupus erythematosus, usually called lupus, or sometimes SLE, can range from mild to severe, and, like rheumatoid arthritis, requires careful supervision and considerable trial and error in treatment over the course of a lifetime. Lyme disease, recognized as recently as 1975, is only now beginning to reveal some of its more serious consequences. One thing we do know about it for sure—it's much easier to avoid than to treat once it has taken hold. The last disorder discussed in this chapter is carpal tunnel syndrome, named for the carpal bones in the wrist joint. This painful condition has been called the occupational disease of the 1980s because it is widespread among office workers who spend their days typing at computer terminals. Fortunately, most cases respond well to rest and other measures short of surgery, which is required for only about 5 percent of the people with this problem.

## INFECTIOUS ARTHRITIS

This is practically the only form of arthritis that can be cured permanently once the infectious agent is identified and treated with the right medication. In most cases the cause is bacterial infection; the joint involvement is a secondary aspect of tuberculosis, gonorrhea, rheumatic fever, or Lyme disease. However, it may also be a consequence of systemic invasion by a virus or a fungus.

## WHO IS AT RISK?

Infectious arthritis is likely to take hold where resistance is low; for example, if you have diabetes or a kidney disease, or if alcoholism or some other substance abuse has impaired your body's defenses. Older people whose joints are already somewhat eroded by "wear and tear" and people of any age who have rheumatoid arthritis are especially vulnerable because the infectious agent in the bloodstream finds it easier to invade damaged joint tissues than those that are healthy and intact. For women who lead active sexual lives with several partners, gonorrhea is an ever-present threat unless the men wear condoms. And as we know from widespread publicity about Lyme disease, the bacteria transmitted in a deer tick bite can cause rheumatic complications not manifested until months or even years after the event.

## CORRECT DIAGNOSIS IS
## CRITICAL

If you have reason to believe that the pains in your knees or ankles or the unaccustomed inflammation of a joint that's never bothered you before are caused by an infection, get to the doctor without delay. You'll be asked lots of questions about recent illnesses and—if it seems relevant—about recent sexual encounters. If you spent the summer on a farm, or you're an agricultural worker or a farmer, the doctor may suspect a fungal infection rather than a bacterial one.

Blood tests are essential for identifying the infectious agent. Joint fluid is examined as well, and where uncertainty persists, a tissue sample may be studied. Because delay in treatment may result in serious damage, antibiotics may be prescribed before the source of infection is revealed by the tests.

Once the infectious agent is known, treatment is usually successful in eliminating it. Specific antibiotics are prescribed to knock out specific bacteria. If the original infection is hepatitis or some manifestation of the Epstein-Barr virus, antibiotics are irrelevant. Therapy usually consists of prolonged bed rest and monitoring the patient for additional complications. The medication of choice for joint involvement is likely to be aspirin or some other nonsteroidal anti-inflammatory medication if tolerance for aspirin is limited. The basic purpose of treatment is to eliminate the infection and then deal with the arthritis.

## WHEN HOSPITALIZATION MAY BE NECESSARY

If the infection gets out of hand because of delayed diagnosis or delayed response to medication, it may be necessary to drain the infected fluid from the joint every day to prevent cumulative damage. This procedure is likely to involve hospitalization until test results show that the infection has been eliminated.

## SOME GUIDELINES

If at any time you suspect you are affected by infectious arthritis from no matter what source, see your doctor at once and follow all instructions about medication. Even if you feel completely well again, be sure to complete the full course of medication as prescribed. If muscles surrounding the affected joints have become slack from disuse during the infection, the doctor can refer you to a physical therapist for rehabilitation.

## GOUT

If you're among the one million Americans who suffer from gout, consider yourself relatively lucky. Gout can be controlled through medication and/or self-management. Also, gone are the cruel cartoons depicting gout as the painful punishment exacted for gluttony and high living. Myths have been dispelled by the knowledge that gout is caused by a fault in metabolism, a fault that leads to the presence of too much uric acid in the blood. The technical name for this condition is *hyperuricemia.*

Normally, uric acid is filtered from the blood when it passes through the kidneys. In gout, however, the metabolic error takes one of two forms: either the body produces too much uric acid or the kidneys don't eliminate the uric acid efficiently. In either case uric acid crystals develop and accumulate in the joint spaces, typically in the big toe. If the condition remains untreated, the crystals may cause inflammation in other joints as well.

The buildup of crystals, which is called a *tophus,* increasingly irritates the synovium and eventually causes acute pain. (See illustration.)

Anyone who has experienced a sudden attack of gout can scarcely find the words with which to describe how distressingly painful it is. An untreated attack can last for several days, during which the toe is hot, swollen, and extremely painful to the touch. The pain then vanishes as unpredictably as it arrived, and another incident may not occur for many months. Before the development of effective long-term treatment for gout, sufferers lived in constant fear of these attacks because no one knew what triggered them.

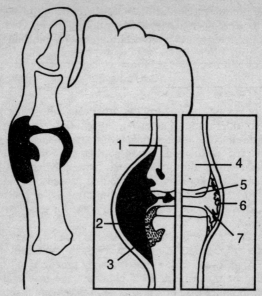

Joint with gout
1—Tophus
2—Uric acid crystals
    in swollen synovium
3—Tophus

Normal joint
4—Bone
5—Cartilage
6—Synovium
7—Joint space

## WHO IS A LIKELY
## GOUT CANDIDATE?

People who get gout may have a genetic factor in common that causes either an overproduction of uric acid or an inability of the kidneys to process it for elimination. The latter circumstance can also lead to the formation of kidney stones.

Most gout victims are men—between 80 and 90 percent—and typically a first attack occurs between the ages of forty and fifty. In women the first attack is likely to occur after the menopause. In many instances people may develop hyperuricemia because they've been taking diuretics to reduce their blood pressure or to control their weight by eliminating excess body fluid. However, if you're in this category, the possible presence of too much uric acid in your blood doesn't necessarily mean that an attack of gout is inevitable unless you've inherited the metabolic fault.

If there's gout in your family history, any of the following may trigger an attack:

- too much aspirin. Gout is one of the only forms of arthritis made worse by aspirin rather than better;

- too much alcohol;

- a trauma such as surgery or a serious injury;

- a diet overloaded with foods containing large amounts of *purine*, a substance known to increase the level of uric acid in the blood. Organ meats are in this category—liver, kidney, sweetbreads—as well as herring, sardines, and anchovies.

## A MAGIC CURE—BUT HANDLE WITH CARE!

For more than 1,500 years colchicine, a drug derived from the autumn crocus, has been used by practitioners of folk medicine. It is said to have become part of the American treatment arsenal when Benjamin Franklin brought it back from Europe, where his attacks of gout were relieved by it.

There's no question about the speed and effectiveness with which colchicine works (for gout *only* and not for any other form of arthritis). The problem is its toxicity. It must therefore be used with great care. An intravenous injection may be given immediately after an attack occurs, or it may be prescribed in tablet form in doses of .5 milligrams to be taken every few hours until the pain is gone—or until there are side effects of nausea, abdominal cramps, and/or vomiting and diarrhea. When these warnings occur the colchicine must be discontinued at once in favor of some other medication prescribed by the doctor. Patients who *can* tolerate colchicine may be advised to have an emergency supply of tablets on hand so that an attack can be averted without undue delay.

## LONG-TERM TREATMENTS

The recommended drug therapy for long-term treatment after an acute gout attack depends on how frequently the attacks occur. Your doctor may decide to put you on a regular routine of a drug that lowers the level of uric acid by preventing its reabsorption as it filters through the kidneys. Two drugs work in this way: probenecid (Benemid) and sulfinpyrazone (Anturane). If you're going to take either of these drugs every day, you'll be tested from time to time for the uric acid level in your blood. As soon as the level is normal you'll be put on a maintenance dosage. The crystals that are present will dissolve, and no new ones will form. This treatment involves a lifelong commitment. If the drug is discontinued, the crystals will form again. An alternative drug treatment blocks the *production* of uric acid. Allopurinol (Zyloprim or Lepurin) may be prescribed for this purpose.

Drug treatment varies according to each patient's needs and expressed wishes. In some cases the two types of drugs are combined. (They are never given for an acute attack; they are prescribed to *prevent* attacks.) In evaluating your situation your doctor may decide that if your attacks are infrequent, you may not need any drugs at all other than a quick shot of colchicine at the time the attack occurs.

## ALTERNATIVE TREATMENT

### Lose weight

In all forms of arthritis extra pounds mean extra stress on affected joints. In the case of gout, obesity may also be the cause of hyperuricemia; therefore the loss of weight may eliminate the need for drugs. But since crash dieting can precipitate an attack, and weight lost in this way is almost sure to be regained, the best diet plan is one that you'll be able to follow over time. If you need some support in this project, try connecting with Overeaters Anonymous or a similar self-help group. And don't take diuretics without your doctor's approval.

## Change your painkilling drug

Don't take aspirin for your headaches or other aches and pains or to bring down a fever. Use acetaminophen (Tylenol) or ibuprofen (Advil).

## Stay away from purine-rich foods

Avoid all organ meats, sardines, anchovies, herring, fish roe, and mussels.

## Watch your liquid intake

Drink alcoholic beverages in strictly limited amounts, and that means beer and wine too; tea and coffee present no problems unless your caffeine intake has to be monitored, and drink plenty of all other fluids. The more urine you eliminate, the more uric acid goes out with it.

## FIND OUT HOW YOU'RE DOING FROM YOUR DOCTOR

If you're on a long-term treatment plan, your doctor will want to check the effect of the medications on your uric acid level. If you're taking other drugs for a prior condition, or you're given other drugs for a new condition, BE SURE YOU FIND OUT ABOUT THE INTERACTION BETWEEN THE GOUT MEDICATION and any other medication you may take. If you've been able to prevent gout attacks by losing weight and changing your eating and drinking habits, that information should go on your medical chart too.

## SYSTEMATIC LUPUS ERYTHEMATOSUS (SLE)

The disease usually referred to as just plain *lupus* is a lifelong inflammatory disease of the connective tissues whose symptoms appear in approximately 50,000 Americans each year. Of all the many rheumatic diseases, it's probably the most unpredictable in its course. Women of childbearing age are its chief victims, and of this group, black women are said to be at special risk, although if there's a family history of lupus, its onset may be triggered in an individual of any age and any ethnic group.

It shares with several other rheumatic disorders the as yet inadequately understood process in which the body's immune system, instead of fighting against disease, turns against itself and attacks healthy tissues. If you have a mild case, you can live a completely normal life, but you have to get plenty of rest and find the right medication (with your doctor's help) for controlling any serious problems. Even in more severe cases, which may involve not only joint inflammation but damage to kidneys, heart, lungs, and nervous system, lupus goes into long periods of remission, during which the patient might be almost entirely symptom-free.

### WHAT TRIGGERS THE
### ONSET OF LUPUS?

Theories abound, but no single one appears to explain all cases of this autoimmune disease. Where the genetic tendency is present, onset might be triggered by a virus or by certain medications. For example, isoniazid, which is prescribed for tuberculosis, and some anticonvulsants prescribed for epilepsy can cause symptoms to appear, but fortunately, when the medications are discontinued, the symptoms subside.

Because women are far more vulnerable to lupus than men, it seems obvious that a hormonal factor is involved, but no one has determined how. In some cases the onset of symptoms is preceded by a period of stress or by circumstances causing chronic fatigue, such as caring for a newborn baby as well as running the household.

## WHAT ARE THE TYPICAL SYMPTOMS?

A major problem in diagnosing lupus is that it isn't characterized by a specific set of symptoms. There might be a rapid onset of pains in the joints of the fingers, wrists, and elbows severe enough to make movement very difficult. Sometimes the ankles and knees might be similarly affected. Symptoms may sound like those for infectious mononucleosis: low fever, fatigue, swollen lymph nodes, achy joints. And yet another symptom might be a tendency to bleed easily. In addition to arthritis symptoms, some women complain of uncomfortably cold fingers and toes; others of a distressing dryness in their mouths or eyes.

One of the first signs may be a rash on the face or neck. When the rash appears symmetrically across the nose and cheeks, and if lupus is in fact the cause, exposure to the sun will make it spread and get redder. This is the rash that gave systemic lupus (wolf) erythematosus (redness of the skin) its cumbersome name. To early physicians the rash had the appearance of a wolf's bite.

## HOW IS IT DIAGNOSED?

Just as there is no clear-cut set of symptoms, neither is there a set of tests that can be considered definitive for every case. The criteria for classifying SLE were revised as recently as 1982, and each year brings some new understanding of how to recognize and treat it.

If your doctor has reason to suspect that you have lupus, you will undergo several tests to help confirm the diagnosis: a blood test for a count of red cells, white cells, and platelets (the blood component essential in the clotting process); another blood test known as the ANA test to determine the presence of a particular antibody called the *antinuclear antibody*, which is found in practically all people with lupus; a urine analysis to find out whether kidney function is affected; a chest X ray and electrocardiogram to check for possible heart damage.

## MULTIFACETED MANAGEMENT
## FOR EACH INDIVIDUAL

Lupus requires *treatments*, since no single treatment can solve all the problems it raises and the unpredictable course it may take with each individual. The additional complication is that it might present itself as kidney disease or rheumatoid arthritis before an unambiguous diagnosis of lupus can be made. When symptoms are life-threatening, corticosteroids may be used at once in spite of their many undesirable side effects. In cases where symptoms are less urgent, it may take months of trying this or that medication to find the one that most effectively suppresses inflammation and relieves pain. This trial-and-error procedure requires great patience and close monitoring. Even if things seem to be going well, re-evaluation of the patient's condition is recommended every three to six months so that any new development—for example, inflammation of the membranes around the heart and lungs or neuromuscular involvement—can be dealt with before damage is serious.

Here are some aspects of treatment:

### Medical

Therapy is likely to begin with an attempt to find the nonsteroidal anti-inflammatory drug (NSAID) best tolerated by the patient. Aspirin and ibuprofen may be equally effective. Other categories of drugs (described in detail in the next chapter) may be prescribed as well, but in each case side effects have to be watched carefully. If, for example, you're given a corticosteroid in doses large enough to control inflammation and reduce pain, you might run the risk of weight gain, bone thinning, bleeding, unpredictable mood swings, and vulnerability to infection.

Good results are being achieved in using antimalarial drugs related to the quinine in tonic water to treat lupus. These are in the category known as disease-modifying anti-rheumatic drugs (DMARDS) and are also discussed in the next chapter. If they've been prescribed for you, you might develop unpleasant gastrointestinal side effects, but a more important consequence to watch out for if you're taking large doses of a DMARD over an extended time is blurring of vision or some other eye problem. If this should occur, tell your doctor at once so that the drug can be discontinued in favor of one from a different category.

You may be advised to stay out of the sun altogether, or if you enjoy beach vacations, be sure to use a sunscreen powerful enough to protect you from ultraviolet radiation. Sunscreens containing corticosteroids, which reduce the problem of the facial rash, must be used with caution.

As in all aspects of medical treatment, lupus patients should never experiment with drugs on their own. If a decision is made to change doctors, leftover amounts of all previously prescribed medicines, together with all other medicines, both prescription and nonprescription, for all other conditions should be brought to the new doctor. He or she can then tell you what can and what cannot be taken together with any new medication that might be prescribed.

One particular problem that may arise: many aspects of lupus and the medicines taken for it inhibit sexual desire almost totally. Consulting a marriage counselor or a psychologist or psychiatrist familiar with the circumstances peculiar to lupus and its treatment is strongly recommended to prevent the breakup of a relationship that might still have a great deal going for it.

## Exercise and Rest

The stability of your condition and the demands of your normal schedule have to be considered in trying to arrive at a suitable balance between an exercise routine and regular time out for rest. Since fatigue, even when symptoms are mild, is characteristic of lupus, conserving energy is an important part of treatment. If you're able to go to work every day, try to arrange for a temporary change of assignments that will enable you to have regular rest periods. At home don't hesitate to ask family members to pitch in. And plan to get plenty of sleep. (Chapter Eight contains many suggestions for the best ways to help yourself and get others to help you.)

# SUPPORT GROUPS

Your local chapter of the Arthritis Foundation can always supply information and referrals for treatment centers, family services, and community help for you and your family. Most communities are likely to have lupus support groups where you can talk about your particular problems, air your anger, complain, provide others with your own suggestions for coping, and discover new ways of developing and maintaining a more positive attitude. Take family members along occasionally, and your concerned friends too.

Information about self-help groups as well as educational materials and other related matters are available from the following organization, for which there may be a chapter listing in your local telephone directory:

Lupus Foundation of America
119-21A Olive Blvd.
St. Louis, MO 63141
314-872-9036 or toll-free 800-558-0121

## LYME DISEASE (Lyme Arthritis)

In 1975 the Connecticut State Department of Health received a report indicating that a significant number of children living in the same area in the town of Lyme appeared to have developed juvenile rheumatoid arthritis. From that time to this, what has come to be known as Lyme disease has been identified in thirty-five states as well as in Europe, Asia, and Australia.

This most recent member of the family of rheumatic diseases is caused by bacteria transmitted by the bite of a tick that lives mainly on deer and field mice. Most people—both children and adults—appear to recover from Lyme disease without any further consequences. But there are some who develop a severe and chronic arthritis as well as a variety of neurological problems that are unresponsive to treatment.

The bacteria that cause Lyme disease belong to an order known as *spirochetes,* and like another spirochetal illness, syphilis, it can develop in three stages if not definitively cured at the outset.

## THE COURSE OF THE DISEASE

Typical cases occur during the summer when the disease-bearing ticks abound in woods, marshes, tall grasses, and especially in areas close to deer preserves and protected parklands. The child or adult who has received the tick bite is likely to be unaware of it since it isn't painful. In many, but not all cases, a small red bump, surrounded by a ring-shaped rash, appears at the site of the bite. Symptoms develop that feel like the flu: fatigue, chills, slight fever, aching joints, headache, and dizziness.

If at this first stage the infection hasn't been identified and treated by very heavy doses of oral antibiotics, the second stage follows about two or three weeks later. Pains begin to travel from joint to joint, muscles and tendons feel sore, and fatigue becomes more intense. Mental confusion may follow. Depression is not uncommon.

The third or "late" stage may occur many months or even years after the original bite. It is this delayed development that may involve crippling arthritis, severe neurological symptoms, heart damage, and other seemingly unconnected conditions. The late stage is the most baffling aspect of Lyme disease.

It is only since the 1980s that what appeared to be a manageable public health problem has become a cause for increasing concern. A great deal of uncertainty beclouds the long-term course of the disease. Blood tests aren't conclusive, and even the rash—considered the most typical symptom and one that acts as an alert signal—is said not to appear in about one quarter of all cases. For whatever it's worth, there's one area of certainty: even though Lyme disease is a bacterial disease, there is no recorded cause of its transmission from one person to another through sexual contact, breast feeding, or even through blood transfusion.

## PROTECTING YOURSELF AND
## YOUR FAMILY

Public health officials are making special efforts to educate local populations and summer visitors in areas where the disease is endemic because of the proliferation of deer ticks. If you live or vacation in such an area, try to attend the symposiums and educational meetings at which health specialists invite the lay public to ask questions and arm themselves with the latest informative literature. Here are some recommended precautions:

- Try to avoid walking in wooded areas, marshes, and tall grasses, and never let your dog run loose in these areas.

- If you go on nature walks, *always* wear a long-sleeved shirt and leg pants tucked into the tops of socks.

- Wear light-colored clothes so that a tick on their surface can be seen easily and crushed by a finger. Remember that the tick bearing Lyme disease is no bigger than the head of a pin.

- Use a strong insect repellent on your clothing and on exposed parts of your body such as the back of your neck, your forehead, and your hands.

- If children ignore or forget warnings and spend time in unsafe areas, their clothes should be removed when they come home and their bodies inspected for ticks when they are in the shower.

- If after spending a vacation in any vicinity where Lyme disease is known to be a problem, you or a family member should develop flu-like symptoms, with or without the characteristic rash, report your condition to your doctor without delay, together with your suspicions about the cause.

- If you wish to have the most up-to-date information about treatment, find out whether the teaching hospital in your area has established a Lyme disease clinic similar to those at the Yale University School of Medicine and the State University of New York School of Medicine at Stony Brook. Where such clinics exist they are likely to be part of the establishment's rheumatology section. These research centers have developed tests for the presence of Lyme disease and they provide instructions for the best ways of treating it. Additional information is also available from the Arthritis Foundation chapter in your area.

## Carpal Tunnel Syndrome

Although this inflammatory condition of the wrist affects more women than men, it is common not only among keyboard operators but also among pianists, truck drivers, carpenters, and hobbyists devoted to golf, tennis, canoeing, or needlework. All these activities require that the wrist be kept in a flexed position for long periods of time, thereby causing the tendons of the wrist to become inflamed. The inflammation is accompanied by swelling, and as the tendons become more swollen they press on a large nerve that supplies sensation to the fingers.

A wide band of fibrous tissue, the carpal ligament, crosses

the carpal (wrist) bones. This band provides the passageway, or "tunnel," through which the tendons reach the fingers, enabling them to function normally. As the tunnel narrows the pressure of the swollen tendons on the median nerve increases.

## EARLY SYMPTOMS

First awareness of carpal tunnel syndrome may occur during the night when you suddenly awaken for one reason or another and become conscious of sensations of pins and needles in your fingers, or you notice the total absence of sensation in your thumb. Or during waking hours you might have the feeling that your fingers are swollen even though they don't look bigger than usual. If the condition worsens, you may find that you're dropping things, or that your fingers are increasingly incapable of picking things up. Your hands begin to feel especially weak in the morning, and the usual manual tasks cause more and more pain.

## TREATMENT

If you have some of the signs of carpal tunnel syndrome, one of the first things you can do is review all your daily activities as they affect your wrist. If your job is causing the problem, you may have to ask to be transferred to work that will enable you to rest your wrists rather than keep them in a bent position all day long. If the discomfort can be traced to overdoing a leisure activity, you may have to substitute swimming or hiking for golf or tennis.

The inflammation and swelling will subside when the wrist is immobilized in a splint so that pressure on the nerve is reduced or prevented.

If this solution proves ineffective, your doctor may suggest injections of cortisone to minimize the swelling and pain. Aspirin and other nonsteroidal anti-inflammatory drugs may be recommended too. And when all else fails to bring your hand back to normal, you may decide to undergo the surgery described on page 66.

# FIVE

# MEDICATION:
## From Aspirin to Gold*

Pharmaceutical companies continue to spend millions of research dollars each week in pursuit of the "perfect" antirheumatic drug, a drug that would not only prevent further inflammation but would also heal tissues already damaged by it. Until this breakthrough occurs, however, doctors and patients must content themselves with choosing among various medications that provide relief from pain and also control other symptoms with a minimum of unpleasant side effects.

To understand the role of medication in the rheumatic diseases, we need to examine the role of inflammation as a normal body process. When tissues are invaded by bacteria or viruses or other hostile agents, or when they are accidentally injured, they become "inflamed"—swollen, warm, red, and painful. Under normal circumstances the inflammation is actually part of the healing process, during which the increased blood flow contains the necessary biochemical weapons for repairing the tissue damage.

At the heart of the arthritis problem is the fact that the inflammation *destroys* tissues, and therefore, short of finding a way of preventing this, we depend on available drugs to

---

*Medical treatments for gout, lupus erythematosus, Lyme disease, and infectious arthritis are discussed in Chapter Four.

reduce or suppress it. This anti-inflammatory activity must be accomplished without interfering significantly with the body's basic defense mechanisms.

Currently, the two largest categories of drugs that suppress inflammation are the *nonsteroidal anti-inflammatory drugs* (NSAIDs) and the *corticosteroids*. The NSAID group includes aspirin, which remains the drug of choice for most cases because it is cheap, easily available, and effective in controlling symptoms for those who can tolerate it in therapeutic amounts. Of the current prescription drugs, Feldene (piroxicam) appears to be a favorite among those who can afford it because it needs to be taken only once a day.

A list of the widely used NSAIDs appears below. All of them ease pain and stiffness and decrease, but do not heal, inflammation.

### NSAIDs

| *Generic Name* | *Brand Name* |
| --- | --- |
| aspirin compounds | Anacin, Bayer, Ecotrin, Empirin |
| ibuprofen | Advil, Medipren, Motrin, Nuprin |
| indomethacin | Indocin |
| naproxen | Naprosyn |
| piroxicam | Feldene |
| phenylbutazone | Butazolidin |
| sulindac | Clinoril |
| tolmetin | Tolectin |

The second category of anti-inflammatory drugs consists of the corticosteroids. These powerful agents are created in the laboratory to resemble cortisone, a substance produced in the body. A brief account of the relationship between cortisone and arthritis might be helpful in clearing up some of the confusion about cortisone's present role.

It is one of the major disappointments in the annals of medical discoveries that cortisone is not the miracle drug it appeared to be at the outset. A little more than forty years ago an American physician developed a substance he called Compound E, based on a secretion of the outer portion (the cortex) of the adrenal gland. When this substance was injected into patients hospitalized at the Mayo Clinic with immobilizing rheumatoid arthritis, the results seemed phenomenal. Inflammation was gone, pain and swelling were gone, and mobility returned. But:

It soon became apparent that continuous treatment with Compound E, now known as cortisone, produced dangerous side effects—sleeplessness, bizarre mood swings, and susceptibility to infection.

Cortistone belongs to the group of natural substances called *steroids*, and because of its many positive qualities, synthetic analogues have been developed in the laboratory. About thirty of these corticosteroids have been approved as safe and effective by the Food and Drug Administration when appropriately used and monitored. Among the approved corticosteroids are those listed below. They are intended to be prescribed in monitored amounts for cases of arthritis unresponsive to other medications, and they may be injected in small amounts for occasional episodes of inflammation that produce immobilizing pain, or when rheumatoid arthritis becomes life-threatening by attacking the blood vessels or the membrane that covers the heart (the pericardium). Since corticosteroids have severe side effects in excessive doses over a long period, a consultation with a rheumatologist is advisable before embarking on their use.

## CORTICOSTEROIDS

| Generic Name | Brand Name |
| --- | --- |
| cortisone | Cortone |
| dexamethasone | Decadrol, Decadron |
| hydrocortisone | Cortef, Hydrocortone |
| prednisolone | Niscort, Hydeltrasol, Medrol |
| prednisone | Deltasone |

Other powerful drugs thought to slow down the disease process are grouped as *disease-modifying anti-rheumatic drugs* (DMARDs). They are described as "slow-acting" since the patient taking them may not show any positive improvement for several months. Because it is not clear exactly how they work, and because of their potentially dangerous side effects, their use must be carefully supervised.

### DISEASE-MODIFYING ANTI-RHEUMATIC DRUGS

| Generic Name | Brand Name |
| --- | --- |
| gold sodium thiomalate* | Myochrysine |
| aurothioglucose* | Solganol |
| auranofin* | Ridaura |
| hydroxychloroquine | Plaquenil |
| chloroquine | Aralen |
| penicillamine | Cuprimine, Depen |

*Treatment with gold compounds is discussed in detail on pages 51–53.

Finally, there are drugs that are thought to be effective against the inflammation of rheumatoid arthritis by slowing down cell division and thereby decreasing the activity of the entire immune system. In rheumatoid arthritis, the immune system, instead of protecting the body against invasive agents, turns against the body itself. But because the drugs listed below suppress the erratic cell activity of the immune system, they are also likely to decrease the activities of the normal cells essential for fighting infections. Therefore a patient taking any one of these drugs requires very close monitoring.

### IMMUNOSUPPRESSANT DRUGS

| Generic Name | Brand Name |
| --- | --- |
| azathioprine | Imuran |
| chlorambucil | Leukeran |
| cyclophosphamide | Cytoxan |
| methotrexate | Methotrexate |

# GOLD TREATMENT FOR RHEUMATOID ARTHRITIS

Gold compounds have been used as injections for treating arthritis for more than seventy years, but it wasn't until 1960 that rigorously designed experiments offered conclusive proof of their effectiveness in keeping the symptoms of rheumatoid arthritis under control in a significant number of cases. More recently gold compound capsules to be taken by mouth have been displacing the injections. Oral gold must be taken twice a day; injections are usually administered once a week at first and less frequently later in the course of treatment. Because of potentially damaging effects on the kidneys, lungs, liver, and bone marrow, as well as the development of rashes, gold treatment is not likely to be undertaken except in the presence of progressive joint destruction unresponsive to other medication. While many specialists feel that the injections are more effective, oral gold appears to be the preference because it produces severe side effects less frequently. Mild diarrhea, however, is not unusual.

Although about 40,000 people have been treated with oral gold nationwide, the exact way in which it works is something of a mystery.

A precise explanation for its effectiveness (when it is effective) is not likely to be forthcoming until we know what causes RA; however, one widely held theory is that gold inhibits the cellular activities that contribute to tissue damage and inflammation.

# PATIENT EVALUATION FOR GOLD TREATMENT

RA patients whose condition continues to be unmanageable in spite of various combinations of NSAIDs, exercise, and safely spaced injections of a corticosteroid, are considered suitable candidates. Before gold treatment is begun, however, other aspects of the patient's condition are considered. Among these are:

- the number, location, and condition of the joints affected;
- whether deterioration of some joints has reached the point where surgery would be a better solution;
- a high-risk condition such as kidney or liver disease;
- willingness to accept the fact that treatment may have to be stopped because of a severe side effect.

If you're being evaluated for gold treatment, you should know that joint damage and deformities that occurred in the past won't be remedied by this therapy. At best the goal is the prevention of further damage that would occur if the inflammation remained unchecked. Also, it is impossible to tell in advance of treatment who will benefit from it and who will not. Six out of ten patients show good results; one or two out of ten show no benefits at all. It is therefore important that, even after the gold treatments have begun, previous therapies be continued until it can be determined whether the gold is making a significant difference.

## HOW THE TREATMENTS
## ARE GIVEN

After your doctor has spelled out the advantages and disadvantages of gold treatment for your particular situation, you'll be in a position to make a decision yourself. If you decide on injections, a gold compound will be injected into a muscle in your buttock. The first dose will be in the nature of a test in order to find out how well your body tolerates it. The amounts are then built up gradually, and when the amount of a full dose is arrived at, it may be given as often as once a week for several months unless it has to be discontinued because of the severity of the side effects. In either case another evaluation will be made to assess cumulative benefits, the desirability of adjusting doses up or down or continuing them on a less frequent schedule. At this time a switch to oral gold may be made.

If the oral method is chosen at the outset, one capsule, or even part of a capsule, may be given each day for the first few weeks until the body's tolerance can be evaluated. If there are no special difficulties, the standard dosage of two capsules each day will begin.

## SIDE EFFECTS ARE MONITORED

Blood samples are analyzed every few months for signs of liver damage and/or damage to the bone marrow production of red and white blood cells and platelets. (Platelets are the blood component essential in the clotting process.) Urine samples are examined regularly for early indications of kidney malfunction. You may be advised to be alert to signs of an itchy, scaly, red rash anywhere on your body, and especially the appearance of sores in your mouth, which might be quite uncomfortable. These latter side effects are likely to be mild and may eventually disappear on their own.

Diarrhea is almost never a consequence of injected gold, but it is one of the most common complaints of patients on oral therapy. If the condition isn't self-limiting after the body has adjusted to the treatments, it is usually corrected when the gold dosage is decreased.

In the event that any side effects are severe enough to warrant discontinuation of gold treatments, one of the corticosteroids can be used to speed the elimination of gold from the body.

In sum, if you're considering gold treatments, you should be aware in advance that these treatments may share the same limitations as the medications you've already abandoned because they've lost their effectiveness or because the side effects outweighed the benefits. Like cortisone before it, oral gold has not turned out to be a universally dependable weapon in the battle against rheumatoid arthritis.

*The suggestions in the pages that follow should help you get maximum benefits from medical treatment. You may be switched from one drug to another in a different category. You may be asked to try a new drug that has just been approved by the FDA. Your dosage may be changed to achieve a better balance between benefits and side effects. If you think you should be taking less of a prescribed medicine, discuss the advisability of such a change with your doctor.*

*Don't take more of any particular drug than you really need. It's easy to develop drug dependencies when you're constantly coping with pain, but instead of providing long-term solutions, many drugs can become an additional problem. The excessive use of tranquilizers, sleeping pills, painkillers containing heavy amounts of habit-forming narcotics, not to mention the daily "need" for alcohol, can undermine your ability to manage your own life and threaten relationships at home, on the job, and in the community. Self-help groups and nonmedical pain management can not only save money, they can also save you from becoming a prescription medicine junkie.*

*Find a doctor you can trust and be patient during the period when you're both facing the challenge of finding the medication that's right for you. If you can maintain a positive attitude, the best available solution is more likely to be achieved more quickly.*

## WHAT TO ASK YOUR DOCTOR ABOUT A NEW PRESCRIPTION

- How soon will this medicine begin to work?

- What beneficial results can I expect?

- What unpleasant side effects can I expect?

- What side effects should be reported to you?

- How should this medicine be taken? On an empty stomach before meals? With meals? After meals?

- Do I have to eliminate any foods or beverages while I'm taking it?

- If I find that my symptoms have markedly decreased, should I take the medicine less frequently?

- Has the dosage been properly adjusted for a person my age and for its cumulative effects over a long period?

- Will it interact unfavorably with any other medicines I take regularly (This should include *all* over-the-counter drugs, all vitamin and mineral supplements, and all prescription medicines for such conditions as high blood pressure, heart failure, diabetes, allergies, etc.)

- Is the prescription written so that it is automatically renewable?

## IF YOU'RE MANAGING YOUR OWN MEDICATION WITH ONLY OCCASIONAL SUPERVISION, SOME FACTS YOU SHOULD KNOW

### About Aspirin:

1. The standard tablet contains 5 grains, or 325 milligrams, of aspirin. "Extra-strength" tablets usually contain 500 milligrams. Some standard tablets contain 6.5 grains, some contain 7.5 grains. The important thing for you to keep track of is how many *grains* of aspirin you're taking each day. (The confusion between grains and milligrams persists because the United States is still measuring by grains, ounces, and pounds, while the rest of the world is on the metric system, which measures weight in milligrams, centigrams, grams, etc.)

2. Find out what your tolerance is, let your doctor know how many grains you're taking each day, and have that amount entered on your chart.

3. If aspirin works for you, there's no need to ask for a more expensive drug. But be sure to take the dose that's effective even during those times when your aches and pains are less bothersome.

4. In order to achieve maximum effect from aspirin, the dosage that's working should be taken at the same time

every day so that the therapeutic amount is always in your bloodstream to control inflammation and pain.

5. Find out by experimenting whether a particular form of aspirin produces fewer unpleasant side effects. For example, you can buy tablets with an enteric coating that prevents their dissolving until they leave the stomach, or delayed-action capsules that release their contents into the bloodstream very slowly. Your pharmacist should be able to tell you what the choices are.

6. The active ingredient in aspirin that relieves pain and reduces fever is salicylate. In therapeutic amounts salicylate acts as an anti-inflammatory agent. In excessive amounts it can be mildly or severely toxic. Mild aspirin poisoning can cause ringing in the ears. Consult your doctor when this occurs. Slight ringing may be tolerable when compared to arthritis pain.

7. If the amount you're taking is affecting the speed at which your blood clots after you've cut yourself, or if you notice that you're developing bruises after only a slight bump, ask your doctor whether your dosage should be reduced.

8. If you're one of the millions of arthritis sufferers known to be taking large amounts of aspirin every day and thereby facing the risk of gastric ulcers, you should know that in December 1988 the FDA approved a new drug, Misoprostol, that copies a natural substance whose function in the body is the regulation of acid secretions in the stomach. Sold by prescription under the brand name Cytotec, it is taken along with aspirin or similar NSAIDs to prevent or reduce bleeding. When it was approved the FDA pointed out that Misoprostol should "permit elderly, debilitated, or ulcer-prone patients to continue arthritis therapy they might otherwise have to interrupt." (The agency also warned that it should not be prescribed for pregnant women because it can trigger miscarriage. If you're of child-bearing age and considering the use of this drug, have a pregnancy test before you begin to take it and don't get pregnant while you're on it.)

9. *Reye's syndrome* is a potentially fatal disease said to be related to aspirin taken by children and adolescents at a time when they are getting over a virus infection such as chicken pox or the flu. If you have a child who has arthritis and is taking therapeutic doses of aspirin, discontinue its use immediately if any other illness occurs. The pediatric rheumatologist or family care physician in charge of your child's treatment should be consulted at once about how to proceed.

## NON-ASPIRIN TREATMENTS

### Acetaminophen (Brand Names: Tylenol, Datril, Panadol, Anacin-3):

These drugs are not a substitute for aspirin or other NSAIDs because, although they reduce pain, they do not control inflammation.

### Ibuprofen (Brand Names: Advil, Nuprin, Rufen, Motrin):

Depending on their strength, some ibuprofen drugs are sold over the counter and others by prescription only. They are similar in their benefits to aspirin, are less irritating to the stomach, and if an overdose is taken, the consequences are less serious than those that follow an aspirin overdose. However, they are considerably more expensive than aspirin.

### Drugs Containing Combinations of Caffeine, Antihistamines, Sedatives, Nasal Drying Agents, Cough Suppressors:

They are helpful for flu symptoms or sinus headaches, but should not be considered for long-term arthritis treatment.

## Over-the-Counter Ointments, Liquids, and Rubbing Agents:

Many of us remember visiting a grandparent whose house always smelled of camphor or menthol or both—and those ingredients continue to be among the staples of the popular analgesic rubs that haven't changed much since Grandma used them for her lumbago. Many of them continue to be locker-room favorites among athletes too. Some names of these products are: Doan's Rub, Ben-Gay, Absorbine, Analgesic Balm, Mentholatum Deep Heating, all the way back to Sloan's Liniment. Except for the last named, which is practically half turpentine oil, the main counter-irritants and heat-producing ingredients in the other over-the-counter panaceas are significant amounts of methyl salicylate and menthol.

When these are rubbed into the skin over an aching joint the result is warmth and numbness in the skin surface that reduce the perception of pain. Since the skin is not penetrated to any significant degree, the inflammation in the joint is not reduced as it is by aspirin and similar anti-inflammatory medicines.

If you find these rubs comforting, however, examine the contents of the various products on the pharmacy shelves, and for maximum effect, minimum messiness, and the least likelihood of inflammability, choose the one with the highest percent of methyl salicylate. All these preparations are toxic if swallowed and should therefore be kept where children can't get at them.

## BEFORE PURCHASING AND USING ANY MEDICATION

To be on the safe side, buy a magnifying glass so that you can read the microscopic print on the outside of some containers and the literature that accompanies many prescription drugs. You'll not only find warnings, suggestions, and generally useful information, but also, in the case of over-the-counter preparations for cold symptoms, allergies, and insomnia, you'll note that many cough syrups contain abundant amounts of alcohol. Aspirin is almost always a component to reduce flu-like symptoms, and if you're on aspirin already, you may not want a double dose. Antihistamines may interact unfavorably with other essential medicines you're taking already.

Before you buy a nonprescription drug, look for the expiration date, which *must* be visible someplace on the container. The ingredients in some drugs have a shorter effective life than others, and there's no point in spending money for a medicine with an expiration date one week from the date on which you bought it.

It's also a good idea to check the expiration dates of all the medicines on the bathroom shelves. If one has expired and you haven't used it recently but you'd like to have it on hand if you should want it again, speak to the pharmacist about whether the original prescription is renewable or whether the doctor has to provide a new one. If it's an old medication you're no longer taking, flush the contents down the toilet and discard the bottle.

## AVOIDING MEDICAL MISHAPS

- Never share a medication with a family or friend who appears to be suffering from the same rheumatic condition.

- If you accidentally miss a dose, don't take a double dose to make up for it.

- If you plan to become pregnant or if you do become pregnant while taking any medicine for arthritis, be sure to find out how to proceed both from your regular physician and your prenatal caregiver.

- If you stop taking your medicine because symptoms appear to have abated or because you're using an alternative therapy, be sure to let your doctor know.

- Don't take the medicine again without consulting your doctor if the symptoms reappear six months later. A more effective drug for your condition may have appeared on the market in the meantime.

- If your medicine has to be taken at bedtime, take it *before* getting into bed.

- Don't carry a mixture of various pills in the same purse-size or pocket-size container. Put a day's or weekend's supply into small individually labeled plastic bottles.

- If there are young children in your family or you are regularly visited by them, keep *all* your medicines, including aspirin, well out of their reach, especially if the containers don't have childproof caps.

## SAVING MONEY ON MEDICATION

- If aspirin works for you, buy the cheapest kind (nonbrand) in large amounts rather than those containing extra ingredients.

- When your doctor writes a prescription be sure to ask whether the drug is available in generic form.

- Make an effort to cut down on the number of drugs you're taking. Maybe you wouldn't need the sleeping pills if you took a warm bath and drank some warm milk before bedtime. Be sure you're not squandering money on unnecessary vitamin and mineral supplements. Try using some of the pain management techniques described in Chapter Nine so that you can do without the tranquilizers.

- If you belong to a union, be sure you're taking advantage of drug discount plans available to members and their spouses.

- Find out whether the health insurance coverage offered by your employer includes an ID entitling you to special low rates for all prescription medication.

- If you're a member of the AARP (American Association of Retired Persons), investigate the advantages of the association's mail-order drug plan. (Don't be put off by the name. The AARP offers membership to anyone fifty or over.)

- If you're on Medicare, find the local pharmacy that offers special discounts to senior citizens.

- Investigate all your entitlements as a senior citizen on a limited income. Many states have created special payment plans modeled on Pennsylvania's PACE (Pharmaceutical assistance Contract Plan for the Elderly) enabling recipients to have any prescription filled for $4. If your state doesn't have such a plan, join one of the lobbying groups working toward achieving one.

- Investigate the advantages of the pharmacy services available to members of the Arthritis Foundation. Your local foundation office will send you membership information on request.

## A FEW FINAL WORDS

With medication, as with other aspects of treatment, you'll get the best results by taking an active role in controlling your symptoms. Check in regularly with your doctor and report any change in reactions to the drug you're taking. Follow instructions carefully about when and how to take your medication. If you'd like to have a consultation with a specialist, ask for a referral to a rheumatologist.

Don't expect the medication to do it all. If you're seeing a physical therapist, do the exercises on your own between sessions. Use the suggestions in Chapter Eight "Helping Yourself and Getting Help from Others." And be sure to investigate some of the nomedical pain-control procedures described in Chapter Nine. You're likely to find that some of these procedures will work for you and enable you to cut down on your medication.

# SIX

# SURGERY:
# From Simple Synovectomy to Total Joint Replacement

## WHAT THE WORDS MEAN:
## A PRIMER OF SURGICAL PROCEDURES

**SYNOVECTOMY** removal of the diseased synovial membrane when synovitis is the immediate cause of swelling and pain in the joint.

**OSTEOTOMY** cutting and resetting a bone to achieve alignment in the joint.

**RESECTION** total removal without replacement of a bone or part of a bone.

**ARTHRODESIS** surgical "freezing" of a joint by a fusion of the joint surfaces. By fusing the bones, flexibility is lost, but pain relief is achieved. Also called *artificial ankylosis*.

**ARTHROPLASTY** plastic surgery that specializes in (1) reconstruction of joints by rebuilding tissues; for example, resurfacing the ends of bones when cartilage has eroded, and (2) joint replacement with a prosthesis (an artificial body part).

Crossing the bridge from treatment with medication and physical therapy to a consideration of surgery makes many people anxious. And since even minor surgery can be scary, be sure that more conservative alternatives have been exhaustively investigated.

For a patient who is over seventy, depressed, and unlikely to cooperate in demanding postoperative routines, or whose general health is so poor that surgery represents a serious risk, the rheumatologist may make a convincing case for adjusting to limited mobility rather than undergoing an operation whose benefits would be uncertain. If, on the other hand, the patient is a forty-five-year-old dancer whose arthritic hip has become a major barrier to a continuing career as performer and teacher, and whose general health is excellent, motivation toward recovery is so strong that the decision to have hip reconstruction or replacement is cheerfully undertaken.

In addition to the wishes of the patient, there are some general principles that govern surgery for joint problems: more conservative treatments, such as osteotomy and arthrodesis, should be considered before arthroplasty; early intervention for the preservation and reconstruction of bones is preferable to total joint replacement; joint replacement should be the treatment of last resort. In all cases patients should be properly prepared for their role in postoperative success.

## REALISTIC EXPECTATIONS

Whatever the nature of the contemplated surgery, it's important that your expectations be realistic. The primary goal of practically all operations is the relief of pain, and in most cases the patient can look forward to increased mobility. But before improvement in motion and function of a damaged joint can be anticipated, the patient's disability has to be evaluated carefully.

Fifty-year-old Jeanne W. was increasingly incapacitated at home and at work because her hands were painfully crippled by arthritis. No matter how faithfully she took the various medications prescribed by her doctor, and how regularly she did the exercises recommended by her physical therapist, she still couldn't pull up her panty hose or do the typing required by her job. When she was shifted to the receptionist's desk to ease the burden on her hands, she couldn't hold the telephone.

Assessment by her rheumatologist and an orthopedic surgeon convinced her to have the operation that replaced her damaged finger joints with artificial joints made of silicone plastic. Although her hands don't look much better than they did before, they work well enough for her to cope with the tasks of daily life—and the pain is gone.

While joint replacement was the best solution for Jeannie W., a different picture is presented by Theresa G. A thirty-two-year-old free-lance photographer, her life has been disrupted for the last three years by the cumulative effects since birth of misalignment of her knee joint. A rheumatologist has been watching the ongoing development of her osteoarthritis, but the time came when Theresa's painful knee was interfering with her work, her social life, and her sleep.

After consultations with an orthopedic surgeon in which various options and their consequences were discussed, partial or total prosthetic replacement was rejected in favor of two other procedures: using recently developed arthroscopic techniques, irregular joint surfaces were smoothed out, and the joint misalignment was corrected by angulated osteotomy. The result was a considerable reduction in pain, and because Theresa conscientiously followed the instructions of her doctors and her physical therapist after the surgery, she also gained sufficient mobility to be able to get from one assignment to another with much less discomfort.

The circumstances that resulted in Joseph C.'s decision to be a candidate for total hip replacement were the following: A sixty-year-old lawyer in semiretirement because of his battles with rheumatoid arthritis, he had already been through hospitalization for surgical repair by arthrodesis of his wrist and ankle. He underwent knee arthroplasty, and because he was so pleased with his artificial knee, he decided to proceed with surgery for the artificial hip. Because of his past experiences, Joseph C. is familiar with the team approach that preceded this type of operation: assessment by the surgeon and a team, including his rheumatologist, as well as nurses, physical and occupational therapists, and social workers.

# IF YOU ARE A CANDIDATE FOR
# ORTHOPEDIC SURGERY

Here are some of the factors that will be considered by your doctors:

1. Do you have any coronary problems, breathing problems (such as asthma), or are you seriously overweight?

2. Are you generally in good health?

3. Do you present any possible sources of general infection such as dental cavities or urinary infection?

4. If you have rheumatoid arthritis, does it manifest itself in loss of sensation in your hands and/or feet?

5. Do you regularly take aspirin or related nonsteroidal anti-inflammatory drugs that might lead to excessive bleeding during or after surgery? If you do, other painkillers may be substituted during the week preceding the operation.

6. If you're being treated with cortisone, you'll probably be put on a low maintenance dosage before surgery.

7. Therapists will evaluate your ability to use crutches if you're scheduled for lower extremity surgery. If your elbow, wrist, or shoulder joints are painful, under-the-armpit (axillary) crutches cannot be used. It is sometimes necessary therefore to perform arthrodesis on the diseased wrist joints before other surgeries so that *forearm* crutches can be used following hip, knee, or ankle surgery during the recovery period.

8. Are you likely to take an active role in your postoperative rehabilitation program?

## MAKING YOUR OWN ASSESSMENT

When you contemplate surgery remember that the operation is only the first step in improving your situation. Depending on the nature of the operation, your doctor will probably prescribe a regimen of rest, physical and occupational therapy, and limited activity. You may have to use splints, a cane, or crutches for weeks, and you're likely to find some of the rehabilitation exercises painful. How carefully you follow instructions about medication, protecting the joint during recovery, and doing your exercises will make all the difference between the success or failure of the outcome of the surgery. Be as honest as you can with yourself. If you're pretty certain in advance that you don't have the discipline to face such a routine, or if your family situation or your job demands can't be adapted to the necessary recovery period, you might be better off with an alternative to surgery.

## SOME TYPICAL QUESTIONS
## ABOUT JOINT SURGERY

### How complicated is corrective surgery
### for carpal tunnel syndrome?

The surgical procedure, called *carpal tunnel release,* consists in opening the wrist and cutting the ligament to relieve pressure on the median nerve. Although this operation can be done under local anesthesia on an outpatient basis, some patients prefer an overnight hospital stay to ensure postoperative care. Following the surgery, a supporting wrist splint is worn for a while, and special exercises are assigned for the restoration of finger-joint flexibility. Moderate use of the hand is usually possible after a week; full use may take a month or more. Regular rest periods are an additional requirement.

## Is there any surgery that can
## relieve excruciating pain around the
## metatarsal arch and ankle?

There are many joints in the feet that are involved in bearing body weight. Following an evaluation of X rays and tests by an orthopedic surgeon, several different procedures can be considered depending on the condition of the joints that are creating the problem. Among the possible operations are arthrodesis, or fusion, of the ankle bones; resection of the bones in the metatarsal arch, and if the toes are contributing to the pain, deformities can be corrected by resection or fusion.

## What is microsurgery of
## the knee all about?

The advances in microsurgery of the knee have been accomplished thanks to a pencil-thin telescopic instrument called an arthroscope. This instrument is inserted into the capsule of the knee joint by way of a tiny incision, and by looking through the fiber-optically lighted scope, the surgeon can make a complete examination of all the tissues in the joint. It is also possible to project a magnified image onto a television screen of what is visible on the arthroscope. By assessing the extent of damage and erosion, the surgeon knows which microsurgical instruments need to be inserted in order to scrape away rough or torn cartilage behind the kneecap, shave off bony spurs, or suck out fragments of loose tissue.

## Will a synovectomy relieve
## painful knee symptoms?

If the synovitis is caused by rheumatoid arthritis, removing or smoothing damaged portions of the synovial membrane is now thought to provide only temporary benefit. However, various alternatives should be discussed with a rheumatologist and surgeon to find out whether other types of surgery would provide long-term benefits.

## What is the difference
## between knee construction and
## total knee arthroplasty?

To achieve the best results in either procedure, ongoing assessment by the rheumatology team should enable the surgeon to perform an osteotomy or a reconstruction at a time when tissues have not deteriorated to the point where only a total joint replacement is advisable. In these procedures the more normal the remainder of the joint and the greater the range of motion before the operation, the better the results will be. In total knee arthroplasty, which has become increasingly refined in the last ten years, metal has been discarded in favor of lightweight plastic for the prosthesis, and the procedure is usually accomplished with the least possible resection of the bone. Total knee replacement has become the solution of choice, not only in cases of severe degenerative joint disease and rheumatoid arthritis, but also in cases of accidents and sports injuries.

## A PROGRESS REPORT ON
## HIP REPLACEMENT

Of the 400,000 or more joint replacements performed around the world each year, 100,000 are the total hip replacements performed in the United States. And the overwhelming majority are a great success.

Attempts to reconstruct damaged hips go back more than a hundred years to a time when various materials were used for repairs. Some progress was made after World War I in the use of synthetic materials to reshape and later replace the entire top of the femur. (See illustration, page 69.) Early arthroplasties

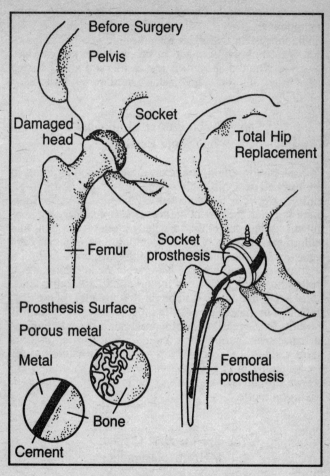

Before Surgery

Pelvis

Socket

Total Hip
Replacement

Damaged
head

Femur

Socket
prosthesis

Prosthesis Surface

Porous metal

Metal

Femoral
prosthesis

Bone

Cement

HIP REPLACEMENT

were not significantly successful in reducing pain or increasing mobility.

The innovation that made the difference was the introduction of total hip replacement. In this procedure the damaged joint was removed altogether, and in its place a long-lasting polyethylene hip socket and metallic head were substituted.

## Some Problems Are Eliminated, but Some Persist

Postoperative infection, one of the most common problems in the early days of hip replacement, has all but disappeared. This progress can be attributed to such precautionary measures as giving the patient antibiotics *before* surgery, examining the patient for other possible sources of infection, and performing the surgery in an operating room especially designed to eliminate all sources of contamination.

The problem that persists, however, is the loosening after a while of one or the other of the prosthetic hip components. Considering that under the normal circumstances of walking, the hip joint must support three times a person's weight, it is a tribute to the excellence of the materials and the techniques of replacement surgery that fewer than one in ten patients needs a second operation within ten years. At higher risk for the loosening of one of the components are those who are overweight and those who continue to run or to engage in strenuous sports.

## Who Are the Best Candidates for Hip Replacement?

Specialists in this field of surgery feel that hip replacement is advisable only for patients who have severe pain and major disability because of arthritis or injury. Age in itself is not a deciding factor. People in their seventies and even their eighties are benefiting greatly from hip replacement. Younger patients who have sustained a serious injury but who have a long life expectancy and are likely to engage in strenuous activities following joint replacement are not considered the best candidates unless the circumstances are unusual. Younger, overweight patients suffering from degenerative joint disease or rheumatoid arthritis of the hip are usually advised to delay the surgery until they have accomplished the desired weight loss.

## Postoperative Considerations

Estimates indicate that following an essential period of physical therapy and general adjustment to the replacement, 90 percent of all patients end up with a pain-free hip that enables them to function normally and enjoy the usual activities of daily life, including a normal sex life. Strenuous activities that put a special burden of weight on the hip joint—such as jogging and racquet sports—are to be avoided. Other sources of potential problems are weight gain, sitting in deep, softly cushioned chairs and sofas, and squatting. High-heeled footwear is out. Swimming, bicycling, walking, ballroom dancing, and golf are recommended.

# GETTING A SECOND OPINION

## Finding Another Specialist

Suppose you're ready to undergo surgery for your knee. The rheumatologist and the surgeon agree that the sooner you schedule the operation, the better. The longer you delay, the more drastic the procedure might have to be. The surgeon says that X rays and tests indicate you should have an osteotomy, that your condition doesn't warrant a reconstruction or a replacement.

You're glad that you're in good health and that you have good insurance coverage. However, practically all health insurance plans, including Medicare and Medicaid, require a second opinion when elective surgery is to be performed. You will therefore have to make an appointment with another orthopedic surgeon for confirmation of the advisability of the recommended procedure.

In most cases a prime-care doctor or a rheumatologist can supply the patient with the name of another surgeon, or if you wish, you can call the county medical society for a referral. If you are on Medicare, your local Social Security office maintains a list of specialists available for second-opinion consultation. And if all else fails, you can call the toll-free second-opinion hotline at the U.S. Department of Health and Human Services: 1-800-638-6833. This number is available to residents in all fifty states.

## Who Pays for the Second Opinion?

All health insurance plans that require a second opinion will pay for it. Under certain circumstances they will even pay for a third opinion. If you don't have insurance coverage but you want a second opinion, you would pay for it in the same way that you would pay for any other consultation. In any case it would save time, as well as your money, if this should be the case, to ask the original orthopedic surgeon to send all your relevant medical records to the second surgeon.

## What Happens if the Surgeons Disagree?

If there's agreement between the two orthopedists about the need for the surgery originally described, you'll probably be sent back to the first one. But what if the second surgeon thinks you'd be better off having an artificial replacement, or suppose the second opinion is that you don't need surgery at all but should be put on a routine of cortisone injections? How do you proceed? Either you can discuss your options all over again with your rheumatologist, or you can get a third opinion.

# FINDING OUT
## ABOUT COSTS *IN ADVANCE*

- Find out whether under your insurance plan you *must* have a second opinion for elective surgery.

- When you know that you have the approval of your insurance plan, find out what percentage of your costs your plan will cover.

- Ask the surgeon's office whether the amount covered by your insurance will be accepted as full payment.

- If your insurance provides coverage for a limited number of days in the hospital, and you've already used up these benefits in a given year, you may have to postpone your surgery until your hospitalization coverage is available again.

When surgery is being considered, the Arthritis Foundation suggests that you ask the following questions—and any others that you want answered in advance. It's a good idea to have a copy of these questions with you during your consultation so that you're sure to cover all of them.

## Surgery

1. What other kinds of treatment might I have/try other than surgery?

2. Can you briefly explain the surgical procedure?

3. How long will the surgery take?

4. What, if any, risks are involved in the procedure?

5. Will I need a blood transfusion?

6. What type of anesthesia will I have?

7. How much improvement can I expect from this procedure?

8. Will other surgery be necessary?

9. If surgery is chosen, will you contact my family doctor; will he or she be involved in this hospitalization and in what way?

10. How many times have you performed this type of surgery?

11. May I speak with another patient who has undergone this surgery?

## Hospital Stay After Surgery

1. How long should I expect to stay in the hospital?

2. How much pain will there be, and will I receive medication for it?

3. How long do I have to stay in bed?

4. How long before physical therapy is started?

5. Is physical therapy/ocucpational therapy covered by insurance?

## At Home

1. Will I need to arrange for special help at home, and for how long?

2. What medications will I be taking at home and for how long?

3. What kind of pain is normal to expect? How long should this pain continue?

4. What restrictions will there be on my activities—driving, climbing stairs, bending, eating, sex?

5. How often will I have follow-up appointments with you? Are they covered by insurance?

6. Will I need special equipment at home? Is it covered by insurance?

# SEVEN

# EXERCISE AND REST:
## Achieving the Right Balance

Scarcely a day goes by when some health expert isn't extolling the benefits of exercise to young and old alike. It's the best way to control weight. It improves circulation, decreases arterial disease, and strengthens the heart. Because it can produce euphoria by triggering the release of endorphins (those "feel-good" chemicals secreted by the brain), exercise is a cheap antidote to depression, and it certainly helps people get a good night's sleep.

For a person suffering from any type of joint disease, exercise performs a special function, but it can't be just any form of physical effort. Getting through an ordinary day demands considerable physical effort: walking up and down stairs, reaching and bending, pushing and pulling, carrying bundles, running for a bus, as well as such recreational activities as piano playing, light gardening, or social dancing.

Aerobic activities that improve respiratory and circulatory function by requiring increased oxygen consumption are always helpful for general well-being. Swimming, especially in warm water, is almost always recommended for those without too much joint pain. Brisk walking and cycling (unless knee joints are involved) are excellent out-of-door pursuits. But these are no substitute for a program designed by a doctor or physical therapist for your *particular* needs.

## THE PURPOSE OF
## THERAPEUTIC EXERCISE

Therapeutic (as distinct from recreational) exercises play a major role in individualized treatment for arthritis. They have the specific purpose of maintaining joint flexibility as well as safeguarding and even increasing muscle strength. Therapeutic exercises designed to restore and maintain joint flexibility are called *range of motion* exercises. (See illustration.) The specific exercises recommended in this category depend on how much mobility must be maintained and/or restored in order to perform such tasks as getting dressed, preparing a meal, and self-care in general. Flexing your fingers, raising and lowering your hand from the wrist, bending your elbow, and rotating your shoulder, alone or with help, may be followed by stretching routines.

The additional goal of strengthening muscles is achieved in two ways: *isometric* exercises, in which the muscle is tightened without moving the joint, and *isotonic resistance* exercises, in which light weights are used under the supervision of a doctor or therapist. Muscle-strengthening exercises are essential for rehabilitating muscles that have become weak through disuse during periods of enforced bed rest because of severe flare or recovery from surgery. Both isotonic and isometric programs begin very gradually, and demands on muscles are increased depending on pain tolerance and practical needs. They should never be undertaken on one's own.

## THE ROLE OF THE
## PHYSICAL THERAPIST

Charles Berges is a licensed physical therapist in Brooklyn Heights whose practice consists entirely of patients he treats through referral or prescription by surgeons, medical doctors, and dentists, as required by New York State

## Figure 1. Shoulder

Lie on your back. Raise one arm over your head, keeping your elbow straight. Keep your arm close to your ear. Return your arm slowly to your side. Repeat with your other arm.

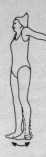

## Figure 2. Hip

Lie on your back with your legs straight and about six inches apart. Point your toes up. Slide one leg out to the side and return. Try to keep your toes pointing up. Repeat with your other leg.

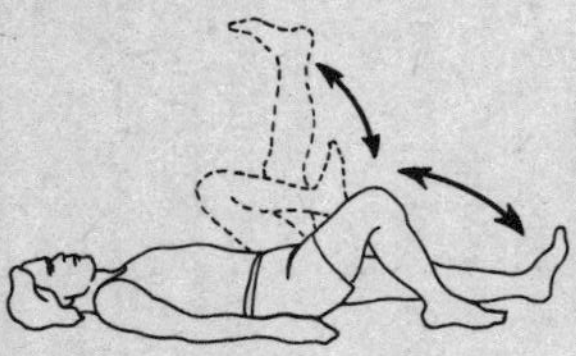

## Figure 3. Knee and Hip

Lie on your back with one knee bent and the other as straight as possible. Bend the knee of the straight leg and bring it toward the chest. Push the leg into the air and then lower it to the floor. Repeat, using the other leg.

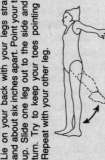

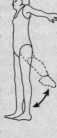

## Figure 4. Hip and Knee

Lie on your back with your legs as straight as possible, about six inches apart. Keep your toes pointed up. Roll your hips and knees in and out, keeping your knees straight.

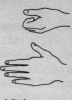

To further strengthen knees, while lying with both legs out straight, attempt to push one knee down against the floor. Tighten the muscle on the front of the thigh. Hold this tightening for a slow count of five. Relax. Repeat with the other knee.

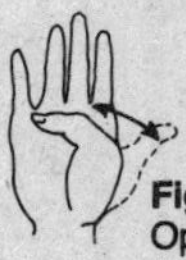

## Figure 5. Thumb

Open your hand with your fingers straight. Reach your thumb across your palm until it touches the base of the little finger. Stretch your thumb out and repeat.

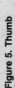

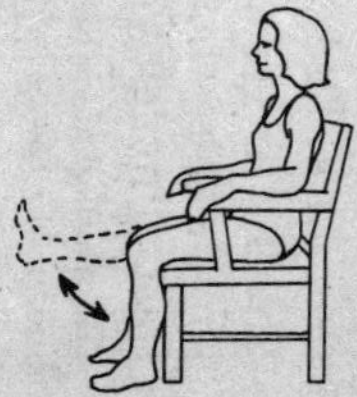

## Figure 6. Knee

Sit in a chair high enough so that you can swing your leg. Keep your thigh on the chair and straighten out your knee. Hold a few seconds. Then bend your knee back as far as possible. Repeat with the other knee.

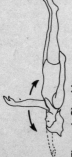

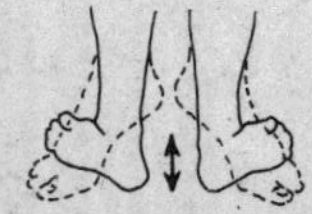

## Figure 7. Ankle

While sitting, (a) lift your toes as high as possible. Then return your toes to the floor and (b) lift your heels as high as possible. Repeat.

## Figure 8. Fingers

Open your hand, with fingers straight. Bend all the finger joints except the knuckles. Touch the top of the palm. Open and repeat.

law.* After he receives a written diagnosis of the patient's condition and confers with the doctor when additional information is necessary, he makes a detailed evaluation of the patient's needs and capabilities. Whenever possible this evaluation is made in his office, but in cases of the home-bound disabled or enfeebled elderly, he sets up a schedule of house calls. These are usually arranged through a contract with a home health-care agency.

Based on the results of tests for range of motion, muscle strength, balance and coordination, sensory impairment of limbs, depth perception, and general mental function, he decides what kind of exercises are needed: both those that can be done by the patient alone and those that require his help. If, for example, he finds that the patient has advanced rheumatoid arthritis and very little can be done to rehabilitate the joint, efforts are devoted to strengthening the surrounding musculature so that the joint can be stabilized. He also recommends individually suitable appliances for the reduction of weight load on the impaired joint such as splints, canes, or walkers.

In taking on a new patient Mr. Berges is especially concerned about clarifying what he can and can't accomplish. "I would like my patients to have reasonable and realistic expectations so that they aren't disappointed in the improvements that are finally achieved. I try to explain that physical therapy is a combined effort, and that by myself, I can accomplish only so much. The rest is up to the patient. The more consistent and disciplined the efforts, the greater the achievement."

He also makes a special point of involving family members in the patient's progress, and wherever possible he will instruct the spouse or other members of the household, or the part- or full-time home health aide, in how to help with some of the exercises in his absence. It is most important for those who are assisting or monitoring the patient to do so in a pleasant and sympathetic way so that they will seem part of a cooperative effort rather than a punishment.

*The states with similar laws are: Connecticut, Florida, Georgia, Hawaii, Illinois, Kansas, Louisiana, Maine, Michigan, Mississippi, New Jersey, New Mexico, Oklahoma, Pennsylvania, Rhode Island, Tennessee, Texas, and Wyoming. In all other states physical therapists may evaluate and treat patients in the same way that chiropractors do—as independent professionals.

Mr. Berges is especially concerned with posture correction. "Many women, especially overweight women, develop degenerative joint disease at an unnecessarily early age because their poor posture results in poor distribution of weight. This inevitably leads to hip, knee, and ankle joint displacement as well as to low-back pain. Wherever possible we try to halt this process by supervising the patient's posture correction exercises until they can be done alone on a regular basis."

In addition to designing an exercise program for each patient, Mr. Berges also provides instruction in the control of pain through moist heat, joint immobilization, and the use of a portable electrically controlled device known as TENS (Transcutaneous Electrical Nerve Stimulation), which is described in Chapter Nine on pain control.

"Patients are usually gratified—and often surprised—to find that their reward for staying with the range of motion exercises, doing them regularly as prescribed, is a marked decrease in pain, and in some cases the elimination of pain altogether."

## MAKING YOUR OWN SCHEDULE

Once you've been told which exercises are suitable for your condition and you've practiced them in the presence of—and, if necessary, with the help of—a physical therapist, you can set up your own schedule for doing them on a regular basis—at home or in a heated pool if they lend themselves to that environment.

A regular schedule means just that—doing the exercises for a specific amount of time at specific times. It's much more productive to exercise once a day every day for ten minutes than to exercise on a catch-as-catch-can basis for longer periods. Nor should you be guided by the "no pain, no gain" concept so popular with body builders. Unless you're specifically instructed by your doctor or physical therapist to continue any particular exercise even though it hurts to do so, *stop* as soon as the effort is painful. You can do yourself unnecessary harm by subjecting an already damaged joint to undue stress.

Most people prefer to do their exercises when they wake up to combat morning stiffness. Many men and women can do certain kinds of range-of-motion exercises as well as isometrics when they're at work. There are those who wait until evening to begin their routine—at the end of a busy day of work at home or outside on the job. If you find it more relaxing to do your after-hours exercising while sitting in a tub of warm water, you may have discovered that that's the best way to get a good night's sleep. But—unless there's a nonskid mat at the bottom of the tub and there are grab bars on the wall—don't do any exercising in the bathtub while you're standing up.

## PREPARING FOR EXERCISE: HEAT AND COLD APPLICATION

There's nothing new about using heat as a remedy for morning stiffness. Some of us remember aged relatives who wouldn't go from here to there without their "hot water bottle"—long since superseded by the electric heating pad. The application of heat is not only cozy and comforting; by relaxing muscles and reducing pain, it increases flexibility of movement and therefore makes it easier to do one's exercises.

Some people prefer to begin their routine with a warm bath or shower. Others prefer to expose the painful joint to a heat lamp. In general, warm and soothing, *not* hot, should be the rule. Heat should never be applied to the degree that it becomes uncomfortable, whatever the procedure, whether application, exposure, or immersion, and fifteen minutes' worth should be enough before any warm-up exercise.

Another way to prepare for exercising is to alternate heat and cold. This method can be used for a hip or knee problem by alternating a heating pad with an ice pack made of ice cubes in a plastic bag wrapped in a towel. For hands and/or feet, immersion is another solution. Two vessels can be prepared, one containing cold water—about 60 degrees—the other warm water, each to be used alternately three or four times for about three minutes each time, ending with a longer soak in the warm water.

## THE IMPORTANCE OF REST

Practically all rheumatic diseases are benefited by periods of rest. But just as too much exercise or unsuitable exercise can cause damage to joints, too much rest can lead to unnecessary stiffness and muscle weakness. During a severe flare crisis, bed rest may be recommended as the only way to reduce inflammation and pain. There is sufficient evidence that rest can actually improve the clinical condition of an immobilized joint or joints.

Maintaining the proper balance between exercise and rest depends on how you react to pain at any given time. Only you can decide that on a particular day you need more rest than exercise because of a noticeable flare-up of inflammation and pain or because you're feeling more fatigued than usual.

One of the most difficult aspects of treating arthritis is that there are no hard and fast rules, and you must therefore be prepared to shift gears frequently, allowing your body to make decisions about how to proceed. And when you're in doubt always consult a member of your treatment team.

## SUPPORTS AND SPLINTS
## AS A FORM OF REST

Weight-bearing joints that are painful need to be protected against further stress. There are many ways to do this: a cane can obviously relieve a hip or knee of the burden of some weight. In more extreme cases a walker performs the same function.

The crippling of some joints can be postponed—sometimes permanently—by the proper use of splints, which provide the support that enables the joint to rest. A splint need not be worn at all times. Limiting use to the hours of sleep can produce beneficial results. (See illustration, next page)

Immobilizing joints in order to reduce severe pain is accomplished with other devices, depending on the part of the body

| Anatomic Site | Problem | Splint |
|---|---|---|
| Wrist | Swelling Pain Carpal tunnel | Functional wrist splint |
| Hand | Swelling Pain | Resting hand splint |
| | Swan neck Boutonniere | Finger ring splint |
| Thumb | Carpometacarpal pain Metacarpophalangeal pain Metacarpophalangeal instability | |

A variety of hand and wrist splints used for patients with rheumatic disease.

involved: a neck brace, knee cage, or lower-back support can mean relief from misery during a period of transition between different types of treatment.

## WHAT ABOUT MASSAGE?

There's no question that certain types of massage and manipulation performed by a trained practitioner will make you feel better by stroking, kneading, and even pummeling to relax the muscles. However, it is generally agreed by joint-disease specialists that these procedures can't be depended upon to strengthen muscles or restore lost function. Your physical therapist may use massage when knotted muscles are interfering with the exercises you and the therapist are doing together at any particular time or when a muscle goes into spasm and causes acute pain. But massage as such doesn't perform a role in rehabilitation.

## SHOULD I JOIN A HEALTH CLUB?

Some people with arthritis join a health club only in order to be able to use a heated pool throughout the year. Others seek out a club that offers the services of a physical therapist who supervises exercise and dance classes for the mildly disabled. Most health clubs, however, offer recreational rather than therapeutic exercises, and their activities are therefore no substitute for a specifically goal-oriented individual program. Anyone under a doctor's care for arthritis should be sure to discuss a health-club program with their doctor before joining.

## IS A HEALTH SPA WORTH THE COST?

Many people with aches and pains extol the advantages of vacationing at a health spa that offers mud baths, saunas, massages, and exercise programs supervised by accredited professionals. If you can afford the expense, a few weeks at a spa of this kind can be energizing, relaxing, and socially rewarding, but don't go off to Arizona or Mexico with the expectation that somebody out there has a magic cure for whatever ails you.

## YOUR DOCTOR CAN HELP YOU DECIDE

Whether you should join a health club, or fly off to a spa, or simply substitute brisk walking for jogging are matters to discuss with your doctor, who will lay out the advantages and disadvantages of your various options. This will enable you to make an informed decision that you won't have reason to regret.

## GETTING THE BEST RESULTS
## FROM EXERCISE

- Wear comfortable garments that don't bind any part of your body.

- Always begin exercises slowly, increasing the pace gradually.

- Breathe evenly and regularly. *Don't hold your breath.*

- When a joint becomes painful and inflamed, don't force it through a full range of motion. Don't abandon the exercise altogether, but move the joint slowly and gently to whatever extent seems possible on that particular day.

- If you notice any change in the capability of movement in a joint you've been exercising regularly, discuss the change with your doctor or physical therapist.

- Learn how to distinguish between normal and abnormal body responses. *Normal reactions* to exercise include:
  a faster heartbeat
  deeper and faster breathing
  tender and aching muscles when you first begin to exercise
    regularly.

*Abnormal reactions* to exercise include:

  dizziness or faintness
  nausea
  chest pains or shortness of breath
  any sudden stabbing pain.

Remember that no matter what other activities you're involved in, only prescribed therapeutic exercises will produce the end result of *strengthening specific joints*. There is even compelling evidence that such exercises can stimulate the growth of new cartilage.

If you find yourself looking for excuses to discontinue the exercises, remember the long-term goal. If the routine becomes boring, play your favorite tapes and records as a background distraction, plan some self-indulgent low-calorie treat as a reward for working out, or ask a friend or neighbor to join you when they are doing their own body-building exercises. Should you honestly begin to feel that your exercises are a waste of time, call your doctor for a reassessment. It might be time to join a support group for encouragement. And if you find yourself slipping into a general depression about your situation, give serious consideration to some form of individual therapy to help you over a difficult time by changing your outlook.

# EIGHT

# HELPING YOURSELF AND GETTING HELP FROM OTHERS

Your doctor has told you that the particular form of arthritis you're suffering from isn't life-threatening, but it *is* chronic, and in the final analysis only *you* can ensure that it doesn't get worse. You've also been assured that, although there's no panacea that will work like magic, there are many ways in which you can help yourself. For some people it isn't easy to be put in charge of their own situation, especially at a time when they're in pain and feeling vulnerable and angry, and maybe even blaming themselves for having caused their condition.

There has been a lot said about "self-punitive illness," and who can turn a deaf ear to constant talk about "stress-triggered symptoms"?

Well, what if there *is* a grain of truth in those charges? What good does it do to add the burden of guilt to someone's real problems of the moment? If you hear yourself—or anyone else—explaining your arthritis by reviewing your past mistakes, you'd be well advised to put those accusations in the category of Blaming the Victim and turning your attention to the here and now.

No one can pretend that it's easy to face the prospect of pain and limited capability, especially when there's an element of uncertainty about good days and bad ones, unpredictable flare-ups of inflammation, and mysterious periods of remission. But try to keep in mind that in coping with chronic illness, *attitude is everything.* It is *your* attitude that will determine the amount of patience and determination with which you take charge of your body and your feelings.

Of course you're not expected to go it alone. You should be able to count on the sympathetic understanding of family and friends. You should be able to count on help and encouragement from your doctor, who can provide you with the right exercise regimen and the most effective medication with the fewest undesirable side effects. Your doctor should also be expected to answer your questions fully and to refer you to a specialist—most likely a rheumatologist—if and when the need arises for further diagnosis beyond the range of his or her expertise.

Rheumatology is a subspecialty that comes under the major speciality of internal medicine. Some of the other subspecialties are cardiology (the heart and circulatory system), gastroenterology (the digestive system), and endocrinology (endocrine system and hormones).

Rheumatologists—the term was created in 1940—deal with the medical rather than the surgical treatment of all diseases of the joints and the connective tissues. Of course in those cases—and there are many—where team treatment is required, the rheumatologist works closely with an orthopedic surgeon. You may also be referred to a rheumatologist by your private doctor for a review of your condition and the medicines that are being prescribed for it.

If your condition warrants it, you should have the guidance of a physical therapist who shows you how to do the exercises individually assigned to you so that you get the greatest benefit from them. And, if necessary, because of periods of disablement, a few sessions with an occupational therapist can provide you with new techniques for getting into your clothes and preparing meals.

It's generally agreed that psychological stress plays a considerable role in triggering episodes of flare, even in triggering the first onset of some rheumatic diseases. In a well-staffed hospital clinic, team treatment should include a psychiatric

social worker or a psychotherapist who can help you deal
with those days when everything looks dismal and who can
speak to family members about sharing some of your burdens.

Some people are helped by keeping a diary to which they
confide their inmost feelings. If you're suffering from partially
immobilized fingers and find using a pen or pencil for any
length of time too tiring, try speaking into a tape recorder
with a good, clear playback mechanism. At some future time
you may want to share these thoughts with others.

## TEAM TREATMENT AT
## OUTPATIENT CLINICS

If you're not satisfied with the treatment you're receiving
from your private doctor, you can call the local chapter of the
Arthritis Foundation for referral to a conveniently located
outpatient clinic, preferably one attached to a teaching hospital. In some large urban areas there are medical centers
engaged exclusively in research and treatment of joint diseases.

A distinct advantage of clinic care (and of only some health
maintenance organizations) is the availability of team treatment
in one place: not only rheumatologists and orthopedic surgeons, but a spectrum of health-care professionals who specialize in your particular problems: physiatrists; physical,
occupational, and psychological therapists; nurses with advanced training in joint diseases; medical social workers and
pain control experts.

Practically all health insurance plans—whether the coverage is yours or you're included in your spouse's policy—pay
most of the costs for such treatment. This is also true of
Medicare and Medicaid for those who qualify for this type of
coverage.

## SPECIAL DEVICES AND AIDS
## FOR MORE SAFETY AND
## LESS STRESS

Good old American ingenuity keeps providing all sorts of helpful devices and gadgets that make the difference between self-reliance and dependence on others for those whose mobility is limited in one way or other. Many of these devices contribute to safety as well as to convenience. The cost of some of the more expensive ones may be covered by health insurance if they can be shown to be medical necessities.

Anyone whose knee, hip, or spine problems result in unsteadiness would be well advised to install bath and toilet "grab bars," which provide firm support and prevent falls. The "Recline and lift" chairs are a much-needed solution to the problem of rising from a comfortable seat without assistance.

A little imagination and resourcefulness can make a big difference in the amount of effort it takes to reach things and put them away. Instead of keeping underwear, hoisery, gloves, and scarfs in drawers that are hard for you to pull open, substitute stacking units with drop fronts that make personal possessions easily accessible. Instead of having to stretch for china and glasses on high pantry shelves, stack the objects that are used every day on a tea cart that can be wheeled to the table. An inexpensive cart on wheels is a perfect companion that can be wheeled into and out of the kitchen or bedroom and bring refreshments, books, and the phone with the long cord—or the cordless phone—right to your favorite armchair so that you need carry nothing at all from one place to another.

Here are some commercially available items that will solve many practical problems as you make your way through the day:

## For personal care:

An extendable two-sided mirror that attaches to any smooth surface by suction cups; scrub sponges with especially long handles for reaching your lower back; a suction denture brush; a nail clipper and file attached to a board held down by suction; a hairbrush with a Velcro handle that fits on your hand.

## For getting dressed with confidence:

Button aids and zipper pulls; extra-long shoe horns; plastic sock and stocking aid; Velcro closings on garments; stretch shoelaces that can remain in place; brassieres that open and close in front.

## For preparing, serving, and eating food:

A meat cutter knife that needs only one hand; under-the-counter jar-lid opener; a lock-in strainer that attaches to pots and pans; weighted cups and eating utensils; a roller knife that cuts not only pizza, but meat, vegetables, cheese, etc.; long-handled tongs that do the reaching; a suction scrub brush for cleaning vegetables; a folding pan holder that keeps pans steadily in place on the stove so that you can stir with one hand; clip-on straw holders; nonslip trays and mugs; a conveniently angled teapot or coffeepot tilter that eliminates the need to lift the pot in order to pour the beverage.

## For leisure-time convenience:

Book holders; playing-card holders; no-hold magnifier that hangs around the neck; giant push-button phone adapter for easy dialing; slip-on writing aid that holds a pen or pencil at an adjustable angle.

## For comfort and convenience anytime:

Long-handled "reachers"; wheelchair trays and beverage holders; blanket support that raises the blanket away from sensitive areas; walker tray with deep removable containers for food, beverages, books, needlework.

These are only some of the useful items on the market, and new ones become available all the time. Several manufacturers and distributors offer catalogs free on request. Two of the best sources are:

Enrichments Inc.
145 Tower Drive
P.O. Box 579
Hinsdale, IL 60521

*and*

Dr. Leonard's Health Care Catalogue
74-20th Street
Brooklyn, New York 11232

Before investing in any device or substituting an improvised or automatic aid for the conventional way of doing things, be sure to ask your doctor whether it would be preferable for you to use painful joints in the performance of daily tasks as a beneficial form of exercise rather than to grow dependent on ingenious solutions that will cause your muscles to become increasingly slack.

## ON-THE-JOB PROBLEMS

In many cases the onset of one or another form of arthritis— particularly when the onset occurs in early middle age—can be traced to the nature of one's work or the conditions in which the work is performed. The day-in, day-out use of video display terminals or computer keyboards while sitting in an unsuitable chair, or of filing cabinets whose contents are almost out of reach, can cause cumulative stress on the joints of fingers, neck, and lower back. Repeated trauma to the hands, knees, and shoulders in operating factory machines can be responsible for premature degeneration of joint tissue. And where arthritis already exists it can be made worse by poorly designed office furniture or ineffectively laid out assembly-line operations.

If you would feel more comfortable from nine to five using a different desk, or chair, or a footstool to give you easier access to the top file cabinet, speak to the office manager. If your productivity would actually be increased and your physical discomfort decreased by an adjustment in the way a machine or tools are handled, speak to the foreman or the union shop steward. If you've decided it's the job itself that has become too stressful for your present physical capabilities, speak to the personnel director or—in a small establishment—to the boss, and find out whether a change in jobs is possible.

When it becomes apparent that there's no way you can continue to market your particular skills without constant physical discomfort and an inevitable speedup in damage to your already ailing joints, the time has probably arrived when you ought to think about another way of being gainfully employed without constantly punishing your body. Take an inventory of your assets. Take the risk of embarking on a new vocation. Go to a career counselor and find out about aptitudes you never knew you had. Use the resources of your state's special agencies, particularly the Department of Education, which administers an Office of Vocational Rehabilitation, or the Department of Labor's Office of Special Employment Services. Consult the blue pages in the back of your telephone directory and set up an interview for exploring your job options—free of charge. And try to make this transition while you're still working at your old job.

## SOCIAL SECURITY DISABILITY INSURANCE

For those who become so disabled that any gainful employment is out of the question, the federal government's Social Security Administration provides two forms of payment: Disability Insurance Benefits and Supplemental Security Income (SSI). The disability insurance payments come from a Social Security trust fund based on Federal Insurance Contribution Act (FICA) taxes levied on employers and employees. Eligibility for these payments are based on the "work credit" established by the employee before the disablement occurs. SSI, on the other hand, is paid through general Society Security funds and is intended for those who are aged, blind, or otherwise disabled and who have little or no means of support.

Your local Social Security office provides a free pamphlet that tells you how to go about applying for either or both of these benefits. The pamphlet is called "Filing for Social Security or Supplemental Security Income Disability Benefits" and you can request a copy by phone, mail, or in person. (It's a good idea to visit the local Social Security office from time to time so that you can pick up copies of current pamphlets that apply to the special needs of you and your family.)

Once you've familiarized yourself with the requirements for disability benefits, you can ask for the application. The information required on the form can be discussed with your doctor. While your own doctor will be in a position to evaluate whether the extent of your impairment does in fact conform to the disability standards established by the government, you may have to undergo a corroborative physical examination— at no charge to you—by a Social Security specialist.

For example, under the "Listing of Impairments" in the brochure prepared especially for doctors, a rheumatoid arthritis patient is considered "disabled" if medical records, X rays, and laboratory findings indicate "persistent joint-pain, swelling and tenderness involving multiple joints with signs of inflammation (heat, swelling, tenderness) despite therapy for at least three months, and disease activity expected to last over 12 months."

Even if the application is finally approved, there is a mandatory five-month waiting period before disability insurance benefits begin. If the application is denied, you may ask for a case review, and if denial of benefits continues, there are further steps that can be taken, including requests for additional hearings before an administrative law judge and, if necessary, before a federal court. Experience indicates that the higher the level of appeal, the greater the likelihood that the disability benefits will be granted.

## SOME PLAIN TALK ABOUT SEX

It's only in the last twenty years or so that medical schools have been offering doctors-to-be any courses in human sexuality. This addition to the curriculum came about mainly because of the attention given to the work of Masters and Johnson. But even though sex therapy clinics now abound— every reputable hospital has one—many doctors over a certain age still have a difficult time talking to their patients about sexual problems, even when they are the result of a previous condition such as a heart attack or arthritis.

Therefore, if you feel you're in need of some help in this area, you may have to be the one who takes the initiative in raising the subject. If your lower-back joints are so painful most of the time that conventional sexual positions are impossible, maybe it's time for you and your spouse to schedule a session with your doctor so that alternative possibilities can be discussed. If you're a woman with a very tender hip joint, you may need some guidance in how to tell your partner that you certainly don't want to give up sex, but you do have to have his cooperation in finding a solution that will be physically satisfying to both of you without causing you all that pain. *The Joy of Sex* by Alex Comfort (1986 edition) is a helpful source of information about such matters.

It's not a good idea to use your aches and pains as a way of avoiding sex with your partner altogether. Such avoidance—or the denial that the problem exists—can only cause increasing resentment. Be honest with yourself. Is it really your arthritis that's keeping you from having sex with your mate? Is withholding sex your way of handing out punishment for lack of sympathy or refusal to be more helpful around the house? If you value the relationship, it's probably time for both of you to seek guidance from a marriage counselor or sex therapist.

## THE SPECIAL ROLE OF SUPPORT GROUPS

One of the most significant developments of the last decade is the proliferation of self-help groups in which people who are coping with a particular problem get together on a regular basis to talk, to listen, and to ask questions of each other, and—what is especially important to the participants—to provide a strong bond of mutual support. It is a characteristic of such groups, most of which have drawn their inspiration from Alcoholics Anonymous, to function without the attendance or advice of any health professionals unless they themselves are experiencing the same problem.

One or two visits to an Arthritis Club—or to a support group with a membership unified by a variety of ailments resulting in physical disability—can be a revelation for someone who has been suffering in silence. Participants are honest and outspoken about their anger and resentments and they also share anecdotes demonstrating how spunk and determination can overcome disablement. The sessions provide a unique form of therapy because time is spent looking for solutions rather than wallowing in self-pity. Arthritis Clubs can be located through the local chapter of the Arthritis Foundation listed in your telephone directory. Other self-help groups for the physically handicapped and disabled—and their families—can be located through the social service department of your local hospital.

For some people the most gratifying aspect of support groups is that the participants not only learn from each other, they also learn to *help* others. If you think your situation is one in which you can scarcely help yourself, you may discover that because you've been coping adequately for several months, you're in a position to be a role model for someone who's been newly diagnosed and has lots of questions that you can answer. The fact that someone sees you as capable and a source of help can be a terrific morale booster. On the other hand, it's a great comfort to know that there are always sympathetic people you can speak to on the phone when your spirits are low and you don't want to add to your family's burdens.

## SUPPORT GROUPS FOR
## FAMILY MEMBERS

In many cases arthritis is a condition that not only affects the individual sufferer, it can also present many problems to other members of the household. Just as there are support groups for the adult children of aging parents or for families of alcoholics or the mentally ill, there are similar groups for family members of the physically handicapped. Some of these groups are spin-offs of the Arthritis Clubs; others have been started by enterprising spouses, teenagers, or a relative who has become the chief caregiver. The Arthritis Foundation in your area can also be depended on for support in organizing such a group where none exists.

## A RECENT DEVELOPMENT:
## THE WELL SPOUSE FOUNDATION

Recently a group was formed for the well spouses of the chronically ill. According to *The New York Times* of February 23, 1989, more than seven million healthy Americans are in this category, and they now have another forum and advocacy group for their special problems. The foundation has already established about twenty-five groups in various parts of the country that meet regularly to discuss problems and share helpful information.

To find a group near you, write to Joanne Watral, P.O. Box 58022, Pittsburgh, Pa. 15209. Include your name, your age, and your spouse's age, and the name of the illness and its severity.

## FAMILY COUNSELING

If your doctor has ordered lots of bed rest, or other treatments mean that you're taking less responsibility for the smooth functioning of the household, don't wait until the family situation deteriorates. The social worker at your hospital clinic, or your doctor, or a community family service organization can recommend a professional family counselor. Fees for consultations with trained professionals associated with family service organizations are usually based on the ability to pay. In most cases it takes only a few sessions to spell out some practical ways to get the household to run smoothly. The essential ingredients are everyone's genuine desire to find solutions and a willingness to make necessary compromises. Maybe everyone's clothes budget can be cut to pay for a temporary homemaker so that your teenager doesn't have to do all the housework. If your husband's spinal arthritis has put him flat on his back for a while, and you can't possibly take any more time off from your job to look after him, you might be advised to spend the money you've set aside for your vacation together and hire a home health aide.

## A FEW BRIEF WORDS ABOUT
## PSYCHOTHERAPY

Maybe you're finding it harder and harder to get out of bed in the morning. Maybe you're crying a lot, or you're letting your appearance deteriorate because it's too much trouble to brush your hair and put makeup on. Maybe you've reached the point where because of all the pain you're experiencing and the pain you're causing others, you think it's pointless to make any efforts at all. These are among the warning signs of the onset of depression, and they're an indication that you need help.

Sometimes friends and family think you're making a bid for attention. "Snap out of it," they say. "Buy a new dress; take a trip; spend more time with your new grandchild." It's fine if these gambits prove successful, but what if they don't?

If you like your doctor and can depend on good advice from that source, maybe a heart-to-heart talk will dispel the gloom. If you need more than that, some form of psychotherapy may be needed. A comprehensive treatment team in a teaching hospital usually includes a psychiatrist (an M.D. who specializes in treating emotional disorders and mental illness) to whom you might have easy access. Through your clinic you might be referred to a psychologist, who is sure to have a master's degree and even a Ph.D. (but who is not a medical doctor), or to a psychiatric social worker who has similar credentials. Neither of the latter two professionals is legally permitted to write prescriptions, but they consult regularly about their patients with an M.D. for this purpose.

Perhaps you will be given a prescription for antidepressant medication following psychiatric evaluation. If so, your prime-care doctor—the one in charge of your arthritis treatment—should be kept informed of *all* such prescriptions and should inform you of possible side effects as well as the interactive effects when combined with the other medications you're taking, both prescription and nonprescription.

A type of one-to-one treatment that is increasingly popular is known as *cognitive therapy,* a relatively short-term method based on the idea that how you think about yourself and the world you live in directly affects how you feel and behave. For example, if, instead of seeing yourself as a useless burden to your family because of your ailment, you can be taught to change that perception and see yourself as indispensable to your family's happiness and well-being, you are on the road to recovery.

## HELP FOR CAREGIVERS

If your spouse's or your own aging parent lives with you and is increasingly enfeebled by arthritis, call the Area Agency on Aging that serves your community. These agencies were brought into existence by federal mandate to provide information and referral for services to the elderly and their families. They can be located in the blue pages at the back of your telephone directory that list government agencies. Look under AGING in the listings for the city and the state. Find out what programs are offered to relieve you of some of your responsibilities: adult day care that includes physical therapy for your parent; respite care for caregivers; escort services, and the like.

If your more or less disabled parent is still capable of living alone and maintaining independence with help from you, be sure that both of you are making use of all the support services that are designed to postpone premature institutionalization: Meals on Wheels, chore and homemaker help, telephone reassurance, recreation programs, and other senior citizen entitlements.

## GIVE SOME THOUGHT TO GETTING A PET

Help in coping with a chronic health problem can come from unexpected quarters. Pet owners have long known intuitively what science now confirms—that a cat, dog, or bird not only provides uncritical companionship but also a heightened sense of worthiness and physical and mental well-being.

Studies show conclusively that pet owners who are hospitalized make faster recoveries because they want to get home to take care of a beloved animal. Stroking a cat and listening to its purr can somehow reduce the pain of an arthritic hand, and there's compelling evidence that having a pet around can reduce high blood pressure, too, thus making a stroke less likely and maybe even eliminating the need for antihypertensive medication.

If you haven't yet discovered the pleasures of pet ownership, maybe it's time to give serious thought to making a commitment to a creature more helpless than you are. Be assured that you'll be more than compensated for your loving care.

And finally:

- See your condition as a challenge to make the most of your resources.

- Experiment with unconventional ways of doing things until you find a solution that's right for *you*.

- Don't let others do for you what you can do for yourself. It's fine to be pampered occasionally, but making an effort to move around is just what the doctor ordered.

- Observe the basic principles of healthful living: keep your weight down; eat wholesome meals; get enough sleep; pursue outside interests; maintain old friendships and develop new ones, and seek supportive counseling if you think you—and your family—will benefit from it.

- Extend a helping hand—arthritic though it may be—to someone who is more disabled than you, and you'll discover that reaching out in order to *give* has many rewards.

- Above all, don't make a career of your disability. Do everything you can to keep it from getting worse, and then get on with your life.

# NINE

# NONSURGICAL NONMEDICAL PAIN MANAGEMENT:
## Knowing the Options, Old and New

What if the medications or massage or hugging a heating pad or a combination of the above don't provide enough relief from pain to enable you to live more or less normally? Don't give up. There are other possible ways of dealing with the problem, ways that don't involve the negative side effects of heavy medication or the possibility of addiction to opiates.

Within the last twenty years or so the problem of pain, whether from headaches or the rheumatic diseases, has been given the attention it merits considering the number of people incapacitated by it. Some suffer for only a few hours at a time when they experience the stabbing distress of gout; others are forced to take to their beds for days at a time because of the chronic misery of rheumatoid arthritis. However, thanks to a better understanding of the mechanisms of pain, not only are new methods available for controlling it; but many older methods, once viewed with skepticism if not downright contempt, are now being used with great success and greater insight into why they work.

# A WORKABLE THEORY OF
# PAIN THAT EXPLAINS WHAT WE KNOW
# FROM EXPERIENCE

Nowadays, practically all professionals concerned with alleviating pain know about and accept (more or less) the gate-control theory formulated in the 1960s. In simple terms, your nervous system can process only a limited amount of sensory information. When there's an overload of information trying to get through to the brain, certain receptor cells in the spinal column shut down as if closing a gate, thereby interrupting the signal. For example, if the arthritis in your knee is sending excruciating pain signals, those messages can be prevented from "getting through the gate" by competing messages from other sensations, such as vigorous massage or ice packs.

The "gate" theory also provides an explanation for what seem to be mysterious psychological aspects of pain reception. A mother running to rescue her child from an oncoming car isn't even aware of the flare-up in her hip she's been suffering from just moments before; a man whose arthritis of the spine inflicts chronic pain when he attempts to stand up straight is so overcome by emotion when called to the platform to accept an honorary degree that he walks like a soldier, totally unaware of his usual distress.

Another recent discovery accounts for the shutdown of the pain receptors: the powerful chemicals known as endorphins manufactured in the brain and spinal cord. These substances, discovered in the 1970s, are analogous to opiates like morphine and heroin in that they simultaneously switch off the pain alarm and activate the body's pain relief system. If it was ever doubted that the province of pain is both brain/mind and body, the endorphin system puts an end to these speculations.

There is still a great deal to be learned about how the endorphins work, but it is assumed that their "feel-good" properties can be triggered by placebos because the recipients "think" they are receiving a curative medicine and respond accordingly.

## MIND/BODY CONNECTION

Physical pain can also serve as a warning that emotional factors need to be investigated. The stress of fear and anxiety and not degenerative joint disease may be the underlying cause of low-back pain or shooting neck pains. Such pains are very real and need to be treated with understanding and insight rather than with tranquilizers, which may stand in the way of the patient's efforts to modify destructive behavior.

We know that the pains of arthritis are often caused by physical and emotional components too. It's not unusual for a diagnosis of arthritis to spark frightening visions of ending up in a wheelchair. These anxious feelings are likely to cause the symptoms to worsen until the doctor says with absolute confidence, "Well, you have a touch of joint deterioration, but it's certainly nothing to worry about." Suddenly the symptoms diminish and the patient leaves the office reassured and feeling better.

## A PRACTICAL SUGGESTION

Before discussing the various options for coping with pain, here's some advice from Dr. Arthur Barsky, a Harvard Medical School psychiatrist. In a recent *New York Times* interview (November 29, 1988) he urged arthritis patients to accept the fact that they have to live with some degree of discomfort so that they will give up the fruitless search for medical solutions. It is his opinion that the pursuit of a medical cure stands in the way of learning to deal more positively with distressing sensations.

In this approach it would be much more productive to learn to use a cane properly than to concentrate on hip pain, or instead of concentrating on the chronic discomfort of arthritis of the spine, to spend time hunting for the kind of chair or car-seat cushion that offers better support.

## THE PHYSIATRIST—
## SPECIALIST IN PAIN MANAGEMENT

This specialist with an M.D. is called a fizz-ee-*at*-rist and not a fizz-*eye*-a-trist. Professionally recognized since 1947, physiatrists specialize in what is called *physical* medicine, as distinct from internists, who specialize in *internal* medicine. Their treatments are based on exercise rather than on drugs or surgery, and nowadays they are likely to be members of the teams that staff pain treatment centers as well as rehabilitation centers.

An increasing number of physiatrists combine their clinic work with private practice based on referrals from other specialists. There are many doctors, however, who are totally unaware of the existence of physiatrists, many who aren't quite sure of the scope of their expertise, and many who don't see how they differ from a really good physical therapist with a master's degree but not a medical degree. However, because physiatrists are enjoying a successful track record in some cases of what appears to be intractable pain, arthritis patients have been seeking them out, and some are willing to wait for a month in order to get an appointment for an evaluation.

As of 1989, there were approximately 4,300 physiatrists nationwide, with an additional 1,000 in training. If you'd like to find one in your area, call the department of rehabilitative medicine at your local hospital and ask whether the staff physiatrist accepts private patients. If your own doctor can't provide a referral, or the county medical society has no member with this specialty, you can write for information to the:

American Academy of Physical Medicine and Rehabilitation
122 South Michigan Avenue, Suite 1300
Chicago, Illinois 60603-6107
312-922-9366

# ACUPUNCTURE

This ancient medical procedure was developed in China more than 2,000 years ago and is still widely used there and in the United States for the treatment of disease and alleviation of pain. The current practice consists of inserting stainless-steel wire needles as fine as hairs at predetermined parts of the body—by no means identical with the site of pain—and twirling them manually or by electric current. Sessions last for twenty to thirty minutes.

The traditional Chinese explanation for the effectiveness of acupuncture is that the rotating needles release energy that has been blocked and thereby, when the energy is released, the body's recuperative balance is restored. In recent years, however, it has been discovered that the sites of needle insertion correspond to "trigger points" known to Western medicine, and that the technique relieves pain because it stimulates the flow of endorphins. It is also believed that acupuncture activates an area in the brain that exerts powerful inhibitory control over the pathways that transmit pain signals. This "inhibitory control" is compatible with the gateway theory.

While acupuncture cannot "cure" any rheumatic disease or regenerate bone and cartilage that have been eroded, it does seem to accomplish the relaxation of surrounding muscles so that the roughened bone surfaces no longer are forced to grind against each other.

According to the Chinese Acupuncture Center in New York, a recent study conducted in Washington, D.C., of over 3,000 arthritis patients indicated that more than 80 percent showed significant reduction of pain, swelling, and stiffness after six to eight treatments. The center also claims that some people with severe rheumatoid arthritis have been able to stay almost symptom-free by having maintenance acupuncture treatments once a week. "Acupuncture will of course not change bony deformities," they continue, "but it is remarkable how well a person can function if he is free from pain and stiffness."

## WHAT DOES IT FEEL LIKE?

The actual insertion of the needles and their removal may or may not cause painful sensations, depending on the patient's pain threshold and level of relaxation. If there is any initial discomfort, it vanishes as soon as the needle is placed into the acupuncture point.

## PRECAUTIONS

It is of the utmost importance that needles be properly sterilized by autoclave, an apparatus that subjects them to superheated steam under pressure. Merely cleaning them with alcohol or some other antiseptic will not prevent the transmission of viral hepatitis or possibly of AIDS.

## FINDING A QUALIFIED ACUPUNCTURIST

The medical profession as a whole looks with more favor on acupuncture than on narcotics as a way of coping with pain, and many doctors have been referring their arthritis patients to other M.D.s who practice acupuncture as part of their specialization in anesthesiology or cancer treatment. If you want to find a qualified acupuncturist on your own, a good way to start is to call the pain treatment center or the department of anesthesiology at your local hospital. While there are doubtless many competent state-licensed practitioners who are not physicians, most health insurance plans cover only treatments by M.D.s.

## TRANSCUTANEOUS ELECTRICAL
## NERVE STIMULATION (TENS)

This is a battery-operated device about the size of a cigarette package, which, through electrodes placed on the skin at trigger points similar to those used in acupuncture, stimulates the nerves that block out pain. TENS can be rented or bought outright without a doctor's prescription and is enjoying wide popularity among the physical therapists who teach their patients how to use it for maximum effectiveness. It has the advantage of putting arthritis sufferers in charge of their own pain management and the further advantage of being easily portable. No harmful results have been reported, but therapists do stress the importance of guidance in its proper use.

## HYPNOSIS

It's only recently that hypnosis has been rescued from some of the sordid mythology surrounding it and has emerged as a useful medical tool in the control of pain associated with—among other things—dental work, childbirth, and arthritis. It is also being used with considerable success in behavior modification, especially in transforming smokers into nonsmokers. Some specialists in pain control feel that it is more effective and longer lasting than acupuncture, aspirin, or Valium, and unlike drugs, it is free of side effects and can be used over and over again by patients who have been taught self-hypnosis as a way of controlling their own symptoms.

Many people have a hard time ridding themselves of all those images from horror films in which the victim is "put into a trance" and appears to be at the mercy of the villainous hypnotist. The fact is that a person who participates in the achievement of the hypnotic state isn't "in a trance" at all but is highly alert and concentrating totally on the suggestions of the hypnotist. Since we know that the experience of pain occurs in the brain, it is possible for those who can achieve the hypnotic state to transform the pain sensation into one that feels more like a tingling numbness.

It *is* true that some people can arrive at a more profound hypnotic state than others. And contrary to what is generally believed, the technique is most useful in aborting pain caused by organic illness or physical circumstance. It is rarely helpful when pain is emotionally induced.

Dr. Herbert Spiegel, a New York psychiatrist and one of the country's leading experts in medical hypnosis, has pointed out that this procedure "is more of a science now that we've introduced the concept of first measuring the person's trance capacity and then tailoring treatment accordingly." For this purpose he has created a "Hypnotic Induction Test" to measure the patient's hypnotizability. The test and the technique for using it have become a standard part of the courses in hypnotism taught to other doctors by Dr. Spiegel. *Trance and Treatment: The Clinical Uses of Hypnosis** by Drs. David and Herbert Spiegel, is recognized as a basic text in this field.

If you wish to explore hypnosis as a means of dealing with your aches and pains, ask your doctor for a referral to a psychiatrist who is skilled in this technique. There are also psychologists with respectable credentials who are competent hypnotists. It is estimated that half of those who try hypnosis experience partial and sometimes total pain relief after several sessions.

Unfortunately, hypnosis is a field that attracts a certain number of charlatans, and since many states have no licensing requirements for those who practice hypnotism, be wary of flamboyant advertising and check on credentials. A reliable source for qualified practitioners in your area is the

Society for Clinical and Experimental Hypnosis
129A Kings Park Drive
Liverpool, New York 13088
315-652-7299

## BIOFEEDBACK TECHNIQUE

The word *biofeedback* entered the language about twenty years ago. Biofeedback technique trains human beings to manipulate "involuntary" body processes, such as blood pressure and heart rate, through mental control and thereby "correct" them. By now practically every physiological func-

*Basic Books, New York, 1978.

tion that can be measured and appropriately "fed back" to the person linked to biofeedback equipment has been subject to learned control: your skin temperature as measured by thermal instruments; variations in your brain wave patterns as they appear on the electroencephalogram, and the changes in your different heart activities recorded on your electrocardiogram.

It used to be considered a fantastic accomplishment—or a form of fakery—when yoga practitioners demonstrated their control over their body temperature or their heartbeat rate, or more extraordinary still, walked on a bed of nails without bleeding or feeling pain. It now turns out that we can all learn how to approximate those disciplines with the right training—training that essentially teaches mind over matter.

Current laboratory feedback technique originated when it was discovered that people can voluntarily produce a particular brain wave pattern—alpha waves—associated with a state of relaxation. Subjects are connected by electrodes to an electroencephalograph, which feeds their brain waves into an oscilloscope so that they can be visualized. When the alpha waves appear on the screen, a particular tone sounds, and it is the subject's goal to sustain that tone by thinking the thoughts or visualizing the scenes that produce those particular brain waves. It appears that most people can learn to produce alpha waves in a few training sessions. In subsequent sessions the subject is hooked up to machines that measure muscle tension, heartbeat rate, and skin temperature at a time when pain sensations are reported. Under the guidance of the clinician, the patient engages in deep-breathing exercises, is urged to think calm thoughts, and receives feedback signals that can be seen or hears audible sounds of different intensity that vary with the rate of the heartbeat. In this way the pain reactions can be seen to vary as patients learn to exercise control over their pain receptors.

## VISUALIZATION

Many biofeedback specialists feel that the best results are achieved with a minimum of laboratory equipment. When patients learn how to get the equipment to respond as desired through the process of visualization, the technique becomes internalized and can be used at home, at work, or before going to bed.

Here's an exercise you can try on your own at a time when you're feeling particularly achy: Sitting up or lying down, close your eyes, tense all your muscles, and breathe in deeply. Then relax your body totally and breathe out slowly, making sure your face muscles are relaxed too. Inhale deeply and exhale slowly as you count to twenty-five, keeping your eyes closed all the while. Concentrate on the regularity of your breathing, empty your mind of all thoughts, and picture yourself walking in a wide expanse of sunlit meadow or lying alone on a sandy beach close to a deep blue lake. Visualize yourself floating in the water, caressed by the sun and cooled by a light breeze. Visualize yourself free of pain. As you create this satisfying situation, your pain is likely to diminish, and when you open your eyes you are likely to feel relaxed and refreshed.

If you're one of those fortunate people who can become skilled in visualization that reduces pain, you're actually practicing a form of self-hypnosis.

To find out whether you can benefit from training in biofeedback technique, ask your doctor for a referral to an outpatient pain clinic staffed by accredited professionals. If you decide to locate a treatment center on your own, you can find specialists listed under "biofeedback" in the classified telephone directory. Have an exploratory conversation on the phone to find out who's in charge, what the fees are, what kind of third-party payment plans are acceptable, and what the price would be for a trial session.

## COMPREHENSIVE PAIN CENTERS

In the last ten years an increasing number of medical centers have established special units for the treatment of chronic and intractable pain sometimes associated with the rheumatic diseases. It is now an accepted fact that there are countless Americans for whom pain is a daily ordeal that dominates their lives and the lives of family members. Men and women suffering from what has come to be known as the chronic pain syndrome often find that they cannot work, that physical activity of any kind is exhausting, that they can't get a good night's sleep. They are likely to be irritable, depressed, and so totally focused on their pain that normal relationships become impossible. Dependency on drugs compounds the problem in many cases. Many couples come to the four-week program at the Mayo Clinic's Pain Management Center after having tried many doctors, many medications, and even surgery.

The comprehensive centers, usually attached to university hospitals and medical centers, use every method from behavior modification to special surgery, and in the process of evaluation the patient is usually sent to see several specialists who will participate in treatment. The first evaluation may be made by a psychiatrist since it is believed that people susceptible to the chronic pain syndrome are likely to have many of the same characteristics: low motivation, poor self-image, lack of pride in accomplishments, and dependency problems. An effort is made to find out whether the patient derives a secondary gain from being incapacitated by pain in the form of excessive attention, withdrawing from responsibilities, and collecting disability benefits.

## BEHAVIOR MODIFICATION

A highly effective approach in treating pain with an obvious emotional content is the use of behavior modification. It has been discovered that pain often persists even when the physical condition has improved because the patient is "rewarded" for discomfort.

Cooperation from the family is essential when the treatment begins with behavior intervention. The patient may have to be hospitalized in order to make a drastic change in established patterns and to supervise withdrawal from narcotic medications. Many patients suffering from chronic pain syndrome take as many as five drugs; 40 percent abuse their prescription drugs; 25 percent are addicted to their medicines, going from doctor to doctor to get prescriptions for Percodan, Dilaudid, codeine. During hospitalization they are put on nonaddictive analgesics and, if necessary, they are given an antidepressant to tide them over the period of withdrawal.

Other aspects of treatment include the use of local anesthetics to enable the patient to undergo physical therapy (in some clinics acupuncture may be used) to do the exercises necessary for rehabilitating muscles that have become weak from long disuse. An essential aspect of treatment is ignoring or discouraging pain complaints and pain-related behavior and rewarding all actions and statements that reflect a healthy outlook and a wholesome sense of self.

For those readers who would like to know more about comprehensive pain treatment, the following is a detailed outline of the program offered by the Orthopaedic Arthritis Pain Center of the Hospital for Joint Diseases Orthopaedic Institute in New York City, the largest orthopaedic-rheumatology hospital nationwide. This pain center was established in 1983 and has become the model here and abroad for similar treatment centers.

GOALS: To enable the patient to cope with pain and to remove the feeling of being dominated by that pain.

METHOD: (1) diagnosing the source of the pain, including psychosocial sources.
(2) developing a plan of treatment that utilizes individuals most directly involved with the patient.
(3) bringing about behavioral changes that would replace pain behavior.
(4) reducing the personal and monetary costs exacted by chronic pain on families, the insurance industry, and the business community.
(5) over all, the Center concentrates on "well" behavior.

LENGTH OF PROGRAM: Total of six months, with first three weeks spent as an inpatient, the remaining time as an outpatient. Entirely voluntary and can be ended at any time the patient wishes. The comprehensive PREADMISSION EVALUATION will act to ensure that well-motivated patients, those highly likely to complete the program, will be admitted.

CHRONIC PAIN: Pain that lasts longer than six months and persistently resists indicated medical and surgical procedures has become "chronic pain." At this point the pain is no longer a protective warning system; instead it has taken on a character all its own. In this situation the patient fails to show progressive improvement and often presents multiple pain complaints that are excessively inappropriate to the original physical problem. Frequently the patient is preoccupied with complaining of pain. The pain has become a disruptive force affecting the patient's life-style, interpersonal relations, family, physical, and business activities.

PAIN BEHAVIOR: If the patient generates behavior that is designed to show the presence of an illness, including refusal to work, seeking health attention, taking excessive medication, anxiety, depression, and disturbances of sleep and appetite—this is "pain behavior." In addition, the patient usually presents no realistic plans for the future.

PREADMISSION EVALUATION: Examination by a physiatrist, psychiatrist, psychologist, physical therapist, and other specialists who may be needed. A social worker is also part of the team that evaluates inpatients. Extensive case history and physical exam; information on surgery, nonsurgery; information about sedative/hypnotic and analgesic medication. Social history; diagnostic psychological tests.

Patient instructed in the use of a PAIN DIARY for recording the times and intensity of pain. The evaluation process takes from one to two weeks.

INPATIENT TREATMENT: After the preadmission evaluation, and upon acceptance to the Pain Center Program, the patient is admitted through the Team physiatrist. The purpose of the inpatient stay is to provide intense treatment for three weeks, during which the patient is examined by the Pain Center Team every day, along with any other specialist who might be needed. Nurses are with the patient around the clock. PHYSICAL AND OCCUPATIONAL THERAPIES begin immediately, and the social worker begins interviews with the patient and the family. Central in this approach is the involvement of Behavioral Medicine, in treatment designed to reinforce the psychiatric elements of the Pain Center.

This team-intensive approach allows the patient to progress more rapidly than as an outpatient. It is during this period that the intake of the patient's medication is evaluated. If indicated, this medication may be modified or terminated.

In keeping with the Wellness orientation, the patient is urged to wear normal everyday clothing and to be as active as possible. At the weekly conference to evaluate each patient's progress, the Pain Center Team begins to initiate a Discharge Plan for each individual. The Discharge Plan is implemented by a social worker.

OUTPATIENT TREATMENT INCLUDES: Physical and occupational therapy, psychotherapy for the individual, family, or with the spouse. Normally, the outpatient visits are scheduled for twice or three times a week in order to receive these services. At the end of six months the program is completed.

The completion of the program does not mean that the patient is FREE of the pain, but is now able to deal with it to the point where personal, social, occupational, and recreational interests can be maintained.

In the final analysis, the ability to maintain these activities constitutes the successful completion of the Program.

REFERRALS: Referrals to the Center are for evaluation only. Once the individual has been nominated by a primary physician, house staff member, insurance carrier, or other relevant organization, the evaluation is undertaken by the Pain Center Team.

If you would like a list of accredited pain treatment centers, write to:

The Commission on Accreditation of Rehabilitation Facilities
2500 N. Pantano Road
Tucson, Arizona 85715

Other organizations that specialize in pain control information and referral are:

The American Pain Society
1615 L Street NW, Suite 925
Washington, DC 20036

*and*

The Committee on Pain Therapy and Acupuncture
American Society of Anesthesiologists
515 Busse Highway
Park Ridge, Illinois 60068

# TEN

# UNCONVENTIONAL THERAPIES:
## Also Called Unorthodox, Alternative, and Fringe Medicine

For the last five years Mrs. A. has been suffering from distressing pains in her right hip—diagnosed as arthritis by her trusted physician. She's been taking her anti-inflammatory medication and following the recommended regimen of exercise and heat, but sometimes the night pains interfere with her sleep and she doesn't want to take any more medication. A close friend whose judgment she respects suggests that she stop eating the "night-shade foods"—especially tomatoes, potatoes, and peppers. Within a few weeks Mrs. A. claims that her symptoms have diminished to the point where she needs only one aspirin a day.

Mr. N.'s X rays indicate that he has what his rheumatologist calls *degenerative joint disease of the lower spine.* His daughter tells him to take his next vacation at a health spa that offers mud baths, sitz baths in curative waters, and therapeutic hosing. He now schedules regular trips to this spa because he's convinced that these treatments have "cured" his condition and he doesn't want to risk having it come back.

Mrs. A. and Mr. N. may be justified in telling the world that these "cures" work for them, and the world may well respond that doing without tomatoes and potatoes or luxuriating in mineral waters certainly can't do any harm. However, here's what the prestigious Arthritis Foundation has to say in this regard:

> The use of unproven remedies is a problem of great magnitude in this country. Most rheumatic disease patients, regardless of socioeconomic or educational background try a number of unproven remedies at a cost exceeding $1 billion annually. This not only diverts scarce health care resources from more appropriate areas but may expose the patient to unappreciated risks. Nontraditional remedies include remedies that have generated some degree of scientific interest or lay press publicity but for which scant data relating to the efficacy are available.

What does the scientific community mean by "unproven remedies"? If large numbers of people claim that they have been "cured" by consuming large amounts of certain vitamins, why isn't that proof enough? What makes a treatment or cure acceptable to the scientific community anyway? From a scientist's point of view, it is not enough that a given cure makes you or me or the man down the street feel better. Such testimonials don't count for much. What is considered an effective treatment is one that after several years of tests and studies improves the condition of a significant number of patients, and at best of practically all patients without causing serious negative side effects.

The most rigorous method for making such determinations is known as the *double blind procedure,* which is conducted in the following way: neither the persons conducting the tests nor the people being tested are informed about the nature of the experiment, nor do they know anything about the control groups. *Single blind* procedure is one in which the experimenters know the nature of the test and the composition of the control group, but the subjects of the test do not. Because the therapies for rheumatic diseases described in the following pages do not meet these rigorous standards, they are called "unproven remedies" by most physicians.

This chapter is devoted mainly to the most popular of these remedies, including special diets, megavitamins, naturopathy, homeopathy, and others. There are, however, types of treatment about which there are many misconceptions—osteopathy and chiropractic—but which *are* within the *range* of conventional treatments.

## OSTEOPATHY

Osteopathy is a system of medical practice that is well within the bounds of conventional treatment, the basic difference between an M.D. and a D.O. (Doctor of Osteopathy) being one of philosophy. Osteopathic principles were developed by an American, Dr. Andrew Taylor Sill, in 1874. Because Dr. Sill had also studied engineering, he approached the human body as a structure in which abnormal function in one part exerts negative influence on other parts, and consequently on the entire body. In this view maintaining the proper balance within the musculoskeletal system—bones, joints, connective tissue, skeletal muscles, and tendons—is crucial for the maintenance of well-being. Thus, osteopathic diagnosis and treatment involves the use of manipulation to bring about the relaxation of tense muscles, tendons, and connective tissue of the spine even when the disease is located elsewhere in the body. Since physicians with a D.O. degree use their special training in manipulation in conjunction with drug and surgical therapy, they are qualified to practice professionally alongside their M.D. colleagues.

Many people with joint diseases claim to have received particularly effective treatment from osteopaths because they feel that these practitioners offer a more detailed and sympathetic understanding of the rheumatic disease process.

Approximately 15,000 physicians with the D.O. degree have been certified and granted diplomate status by the National Board of Osteopathic Examiners, founded in 1935. These practitioners are licensed to practice in all but three states nationwide, the exceptions being Louisiana, North Carolina, and Texas.

If you wish to connect with a qualified doctor of osteopathy in your area and can't locate one through the classified listings in your phonebook, write to the:

National Board of Osteopathic Medical Examiners
2700 River Road, Suite 407
Des Plaines, IL 60018
312-635-9955

If an osteopathic practitioner has been recommended by a friend, keep in mind that there are no licensed lay osteopaths in the United States as there are in Great Britain, and when you call to make an appointment for a consultation, be sure to ask whether the practitioner is a board-certified physician with hospital connections.

## CHIROPRACTIC

Manipulation as a form of "healing" has an ancient history that can be traced to the Babylonians and Egyptians. But it wasn't until a Canadian "healer" named David Palmer restored the hearing of a workman deaf for seventeen years by manipulating his neck that the modern discipline of chiropractic was born. The event occurred in 1895. The term *chiropractic*—from the Greek words *cheir,* meaning "hand," and *praktikos,* meaning "done by"—was coined soon after, and from that time to this the method has inspired enthusiastic support and strong opposition.

The theory on which Palmer evolved his hands-on system was based on the principle that the unimpeded functioning of the nervous system was the foundation of human health. Any impediment to the free flow of nervous impulses was therefore the cause of malfunction. In his terminology such an impediment was the result of "subluxation," or a dislocation of one or more of the spinal vertebrae. Palmer was able to point to the restoration of the workman's hearing through manipulation of the cervical vertebrae in a way that reestablished the free flow of the impulses carried by the auditory nerve from the upper spine to the brain.

While most contemporary chiropractors have discarded the "single cause, single cure" approach of Palmer, there remain those few who take an adversarial role vis à vis the multifaceted approach of conventional medical practice, and it is these ideologists whose extravagant claims keep the fires of controversy burning. This group, small but highly vocal, has its fanatical supporters who claim that manipulation of the spine can cure everything from depression to a diseased pancreas.

A considerably larger number of chiropractors—an estimated 10 percent of the approximately 25,000 practitioners licensed in all fifty states—describe themselves as "holistic" therapists, making recommendations about nutrition, vitamin supplements, meditation, or psychotherapy. These are known as "mixers," and they usually attempt to re-educate their patients about preventive care so that they can maintain good health without medication. While they are not permitted to advertise themselves as diagnosticians who treat diseases, many of their patients prefer them to conventional physicians.

In contrast, the majority of present-day chiropractors are known as "straights" because their chief concern is to discover the site of the derangements in the patient's spine and, by manipulation and "adjustment" of the subluxation, restore the balance of the neuroskeletal structure, thereby assuring that nerve impulses can flow freely through unobstructed channels. No matter what their basic philosophy, chiropractors may not prescribe drugs or perform surgery.

There are at least twenty colleges of chiropractic in the United States, none of which is accredited by an evaluating body outside of the profession. Only some of them are accredited by the council on Chiropractic Education. These colleges offer an increasingly broad-based curriculum in the biomedical sciences in addition to specialized training in manipulation technique. The profession has achieved recognition by the Federal Department of Health and Human Services, and chiropractic treatment is now included in the coverage of Medicare, Medicaid, and other health insurance plans.

While the official position of the American Medical Association continues to be that chiropractic may do more harm than good, it is not unusual for a physician to refer a patient with a neck or lower back problem to a chiropractor. Also, the profession is expanding and enjoying a renewed popularity, thanks to the involvement of more and more men and women in active sports and body building, activities in which there is an abundance of accidents and injuries affecting the musculoskeletal system.

## ARTHRITIS AND CHIROPRACTIC

If your prime-care physician refers you to a chiropractor for evaluation and treatment, the diagnosis of your condition is likely to be based not only on your medical history and a detailed examination of your spine and the rest of your skeleton but also on posture analysis, X rays, and an electrocardiogram. And if you are being treated by a chiropractor through a referral, then your prime-care doctor remains in charge of your case and should receive regular reports from the chiropractor.

If, on the other hand, like countless arthritis sufferers, you decide to go to a particular chiropractor on a friend's recommendation, or you locate one on your own, you will have to take the responsibility of deciding whether you're being helped. Since many people with one of the rheumatic diseases may suffer not so much from the destruction of cartilage and bone but because of muscle spasms and increasingly faulty aligments in the affected area, manipulation may provide some relief. However, in advanced cases of joint destruction, there is little or no likelihood that manipulation can bring about any improvement. It is therefore unlikely that a responsible chiropractor would hold out the promise of a "cure" for such a condition.

## DIET

The relationship between diet—the collective term for the foods we eat—and disease has been in the forefront of the news for a long time. While too many Americans continue to consume too many greasy hamburgers and french fries and to use too much salt, more and more people are making an effort to eat more sensibly, thereby reducing the risk of stroke, heart attack, and certain kinds of cancer. As for the effect of particular foods on the rheumatic diseases, it is now known that while gluttony and high living are not the cause of gout, diet does play a role in controlling it.* It is also increasingly accepted even among conservative rheumatologists that

> ... rheumatic symptoms might reflect allergic hypersensitivity in the same manner as more traditionally recognized forms of food allergies, such as eczema, urticaria, asthma, and gastrointestinal problems. ... Our traditional view that patients with rheumatic diseases should follow a sound, balanced diet and that no further relationship exists between food and clinical symptoms is changing. Provocative experimental and clinical observations suggest that nutritional modulation might affect autoimmunity and clinical disease. Further, certain patients may have found food sensitivity as the basis for their symptoms. These concepts should be considered potentially exciting hypotheses that are now undergoing experimental testing.**

This statement, tentative though it is, can be translated to mean "Yes, what you eat *can* affect the course of your condition." As matters now stand, however, it is impossible, for example, to say about a particular diet—as one can say about aspirin—that there is unambiguous evidence of its beneficial effects in most cases of arthritis. Still, there is enough evidence from enough reliable people that an alteration in their food habits brought about a decrease in inflammation and pain.

It is unfortunate that food faddists have confused the issue by their extravagant and unsubstantiated claims about "natural" and "organically grown" foods, claims that serve no better purpose than to make heaps of money for so-called health-food stores.

Nor is there agreement even among doctors and nutritionists who recommend dietary therapy for rheumatic diseases.

*See Chapter Four.
**Primer in the Rheumatic Diseases* publ. by the Arthritis Foundation, Atlanta, Georgia, 9th edition, 1988.

Some doctors, for example, promote a diet that concentrates on seafood and vegetables and eliminates all meat, all fruit, and all dairy products, including yogurt. They also warn against all additives, preservatives, and chemicals.

Another diet sponsored by some nutritionists for its benefits to arthritis sufferers is essentially the same as the one that has become increasingly popular with vegetarians: very high in fish content, complex carbohydrates, and fiber, and very low in animal fat, which means that skim milk and yogurt are fine, but hard cheeses and egg yolks are not.

As someone coping with arthritis, you may have discovered that certain fruits and vegetables produce adverse effects, especially those belonging to the nightshade family: tomatoes, purple eggplant, all varieties of peppers, and white potatoes. But if you're going to experiment on your own to find out which foods trigger episodes of inflammation, be as orderly as you can about keeping notes. It's pretty simple, for example, to conclude that you're sensitive to MSG (monosodium glutenate) if every time you eat in a Chinese restaurant you develop a terrible headache. But how can you find out whether a particular flare-up in your hands or your hip was caused by the egg in the mayonnaise dressing, or by the fresh pineapple, or whether it should be attributed to a change in the weather, or to a stressful spat you had with your spouse?

One way to find out is to keep a food diary. If you think a particular food or food group is triggering pains in your joints, eliminate it from your diet for several days. If those days are free of special discomfort, reintroduce the food or foods, and if within eight hours you're experiencing more pain than usual, there's probably a cause-and-effect relationship.

You may be doing yourself some good in running these tests on your own, but if in the process you find you're eliminating some basic nutrients and using heavy vitamin supplements to compensate for the nutritional loss, it's time to discuss your dietary experiments with your prime-care doctor. A correctly balanced vegetarian diet, for example, can do people with arthritis more good than harm, but the same can't be said for certain kinds of trendy cure-all "macrobiotic" diets that are likely to leave the improperly informed enthusiast with a nutritional deficiency.

## MEGAVITAMINS AND MINERAL SUPPLEMENTS

While even the most conservative doctor is not likely to see any harm in your taking a daily multivitamin/mineral supplement, most doctors take a dim view of self-medication with megavitamins, especially in the absence of periodic checkups to find out about their effects. It's no secret that the jury is still out—and is likely to remain out for the foreseeable future—on the relative benefits of a nutritionally balanced diet when compared to selective food choices augmented with doses of vitamins and minerals. In trying to make sense of this ongoing debate, anyone embarking on this form of therapy as a way of halting the progress of joint disease would be wise to separate fact from fiction and faddism from reliable (more or less) information. Keep in mind that it is beyond the scope of this book to evaluate the role of vitamin and mineral therapy in preventing or curing such diseases as cancer, schizophrenia, alcoholism, atherosclerosis, and the common cold. And this would appear to be the place to stress that while some people suffer from both osteoporosis *and* osteoarthritis, no direct connection has been established between the two conditions. Thus, whatever therapy you've devised for coping with or preventing osteoporosis is not likely to affect a rheumatic condition.

There's no doubt that people who are in pain and facing the prospect of increasingly limited mobility will turn to unorthodox therapies in desperation. Others see no harm—and hope for possible benefits—when they experiment with certain fringe treatments. Still others become true believers because after a week of megavitamins and zinc, their symptoms seemed to vanish. What they won't concede is that, given the unpredictable nature of arthritis, their symptoms might have gone into remission anyway.

If you're going to turn to an expert in this alternative therapy—either a self-styled expert or one with professional credentials—you needn't accept the advice you're given as gospel. However, when you're in doubt you have to ask the right questions in order to get the right answers, and you can ask meaningful questions only if you've provided yourself with some basic information. Hence the charts on pages 126–35.

## WHAT ARE THE BOUNDARIES OF SAFETY?

Recommended dietary allowances (RDAs) based on available scientific knowledge have been established for essential nutrients by the Food and Nutrition Board of the National Academy of Sciences National Research Council. These RDA recommendations vary in terms of sex and age. For the sake of convenience in food labeling, the RDA recommendations are set by the U.S. Food and Drug Administration as a single number without regard to these variables.

The tables that follow indicate accepted standards and the dangers of overdose. What constitutes overdose remains open to question. Some traditional nutritionists define as excessive any amount that is twice or three times the recommended amount for minerals and most vitamins. However, because vitamins A and D can be dangerous even in small amounts in excess of those recommended, they must be approached with considerably more caution. It is for this reason that the American Medical Association considers the prescription of megadoses of vitamin A for osteoarthritis to be a flagrant example of vitamin misuse.

Proponents of vitamin C megadoses as treatment for several of the rheumatic diseases, especially for rheumatoid arthritis, respond to critics by pointing out that there's no possible harm in this treatment since the body can't handle any more than 100 milligrams of vitamin C a day anyway. The rest is eliminated in the urine. But what these proponents don't take into account is that when the body has become accustomed to large amounts of vitamin C, trying to go back to normal amounts can cause symptoms of scurvy—

## VITAMIN FACTS

| Vitamins | U.S. RDA for Adults and Children Over Four | Some Significant Sources | Some Major Physiological Functions | Some Deficiency Symptoms | Some Overconsumption Symptoms |
|---|---|---|---|---|---|
| **FAT-SOLUBLE VITAMINS** | | | | | |
| **VITAMIN A** (*retinol, provitamin carotenoids*) | 5,000 IU | *Retinol:* liver, butter, whole milk, cheese, egg yolk. *Provitamin A:* carrots, leafy green vegetables, sweet potatoes, pumpkin, winter squash, apricots, cantaloupe, fortified margarine. | Assists formation and maintenance of skin and mucous membranes, thus increasing resistance to infections. Functions in visual processes and forms visual purple. Promotes bone and tooth development. | Mild: night-blindness, diarrhea, intestinal infections, impaired growth. Severe: xerophthalmia. | Mild: nausea, irritability, blurred vision. Severe: growth retardation, enlargement of liver and spleen, loss of hair, rheumatic pain, increased pressure in skull, dermal changes. |
| **VITAMIN D** (*calciferol*) | 400 IU | Vitamin D fortified dairy products; fortified margarine; fish oils; egg yolk. Synthesized by sunlight action on skin. | Promotes ossification of bones and teeth, increases intestinal absorption of calcium. | Rickets in children; osteomalacia in adults, rare. | Mild: nausea, weight loss, irritability. Severe: mental and physical growth retardation, kidney damage, mobilization of calcium from bony tissue and deposition in soft tissues. |

| | | Sources | Functions | Deficiency | Toxicity/Megadose |
|---|---|---|---|---|---|
| **VITAMIN E** *(tocopherol)* | 30 IU | Vegetable oil, margarine, shortening; green and leafy vegetables; wheat germ, whole grain products; egg yolk; butter, liver. | Functions as antioxidant protecting vitamins A and C and fatty acids from destruction; and prevents cell-membrane damage. | Almost impossible to produce without starvation; possible anemia in low-birth-weight infants. | Nontoxic under normal conditions. |

WATER-SOLUBLE VITAMINS

| | | Sources | Functions | Deficiency | Toxicity/Megadose |
|---|---|---|---|---|---|
| **VITAMIN C** *(ascorbic acid)* | 60 mg | Broccoli, sweet and hot peppers, collards, brussels sprouts, strawberries, orange, kale, grapefruit, papaya, potato, mango, tangerine, spinach, tomato. | Forms cementing substances, such as collagen, that hold body cells together, thus strengthening blood vessels, hastening healing of wounds and bones, and increasing resistance to infection. Aids in use of iron. | Mild: bruise easily, bleeding gums. Severe: scurvy. | When megadose is discontinued, deficiency symptoms may briefly appear until the body adapts. Newborns whose mothers took megadoses will show deficiency symptoms after birth until the body adapts. |
| **THIAMIN** *(vitamin B₁)* | 1.5 mg | Pork, liver, meat; whole grains, fortified grain products; legumes; nuts. | Functions as part of a coenzyme to promote carbohydrate metabolism, production of ribose, a constituent of DNA and RNA. Promotes normal appetite and normal functioning of nervous system. | Impaired growth, wasting of tissues, mental confusion, low morale, edema. Severe: beriberi. | None reported. |

| Vitamins | U.S. RDA for Adults and Children Over Four | Some Significant Sources | Some Major Physiological Functions | Some Deficiency Symptoms | Some Overconsumption Symptoms |
|---|---|---|---|---|---|
| **RIBOFLAVIN** *(vitamin B₂)* | 1.7 mg | Liver; milk, yogurt, cottage cheese; meat; fortified grain products. | Functions as part of a coenzyme assisting cells to use oxygen for the release of energy from food. Promotes good vision and healthy skin. | Lesions of cornea, cracks at corners of mouth. | None reported. |
| **NIACIN** *(nicotinamide, nicotinic acid)* | 20 mg | Liver, meat, poultry, fish; peanuts; fortified grain products. Synthesized from tryptophan (on the average 1 mg of niacin from 60 mg of dietary tryptophan). | Functions as part of a coenzyme in fat synthesis, tissue respiration, and utilization of carbohydrate for energy. Promotes healthy skin, nerves, and digestive tract. Aids digestion and fosters normal appetite. | Skin and gastrointestinal lesions, anorexia, weakness, irritability, vertigo. Severe: pellagra. | None reported for nicotinamide. Flushing, headache, cramps, nausea for nicotinic acid. |

| | Amount | Sources | Functions | Deficiency | Excess |
|---|---|---|---|---|---|
| **FOLACIN** *(folic acid)* | 0.4 mg | Liver; legumes; green leafy vegetables. | Functions as part of coenzymes in amino acid and nucleoprotein metabolism. Promotes red blood cell formation. | Red tongue, diarrhea, anemia. | May obscure the existence of pernicious anemia. |
| **VITAMIN B6** *(pyridoxine, pyridoxal, pyridoxamine)* | 2.0 mg | Meat, poultry, fish, shellfish; green and leafy vegetables; whole grains, legumes. | Functions as part of a coenzyme involved in protein metabolism, assists in conversion of tryptophan to niacin, fatty acid metabolism, and red blood cell formation. | Irritability, muscle twitching, dermatitis near eyes, kidney stones, hypochromic anemia. | None reported |
| **VITAMIN B12** | 6.0 mcg | Meat, poultry, fish, shellfish; eggs; milk and milk products. | Functions in coenzymes involved in nucleic acid synthesis and biological methylation. Assists in development of normal red blood cells and maintenance of nerve tissue. | Severe: pernicious anemia, neurological disorders. | None reported |

| Vitamins | U.S. RDA for Adults and Children Over Four | Some Significant Sources | Some Major Physiological Functions | Some Deficiency Symptoms | Some Overconsumption Symptoms |
|---|---|---|---|---|---|
| BIOTIN | 0.3 mg | Kidney, liver, milk; egg yoke; most fresh vegetables | Functions as part of a coenzyme involved in fat synthesis, amino acid metabolism, and glycogen formation. | Fatigue, depression, nausea, dermatitis, muscular pains. | None reported. |
| PANTOTHENIC ACID | 10 mg | Liver, kidney, meats; milk; egg yolk; whole grains; legumes. | Functions as part of a coenzyme involved in energy metabolism. | Rare because found in most foods. Fatigue, sleep disturbances, nausea. | None reported. |

## MINERAL FACTS

| Nutrient | RDA for Adults and Children Over Four[a] | Some Significant Sources | Some Major Physiological Functions | Some Deficiency Symptoms | Some Overconsumption Symptoms |
|---|---|---|---|---|---|
| | | MACROMINERALS | | | |
| CALCIUM | 1,000 to 1,500 mg[b] | Milk and milk products, green leafy vegetables, citrus fruits, dried peas and beans, sardines and shellfish. | Helps build strong bones and teeth. Helps blood clot. Helps muscles and nerves function normally. Needed to activate certain enzymes which help change food into energy. | Rickets in children; osteoporosis in adults. | Drowsiness, calcium deposits. |
| PHOSPHORUS | 1,000 mg | Meat, poultry, fish, eggs, dried peas and beans, milk and milk products, egg yolk, and whole-grain bread and cereal. | With calcium, helps build strong bones and teeth. Needed by certain enzymes which help change food into energy. | Weakness, bone pain, decreased appetite (rare). | Upset of the calcium-phosphorus ratio, hindering uptake of calcium. |

[a]The RDA ranges, established by the Food and Nutrition Board of the National Academy of Sciences National Research Council, are for healthy people. The lower figures represent the RDA for children, the higher figures are the maximum for adults and should not be exceeded since the toxic levels may not be much higher.

[b]The RDA for calcium is under study. This is the amount now recommended by the Food and Drug Administration and is higher than the former RDA.

| Nutrient | RDA for Adults and Children Over Four[a] | Some Significant Sources | Some Major Physiological Functions | Some Deficiency Symptoms | Some Overconsumption Symptoms |
|---|---|---|---|---|---|
| SODIUM | 450 to 3,300 mg | Processed foods, ham, meat, fish, poultry, eggs, milk. | Helps maintain water balance inside and outside cells. | Water retention (edema); loss of sodium through extreme perspiration can cause muscle cramps, headache, weakness. | High blood pressure, kidney disease, cirrhosis of the liver, congestive heart disease. |
| CHLORIDE | 700 to 5,100 mg | Table salt, same as sodium. | Part of hydrochloric acid found in gastric juice and important to normal digestion. | Upset balance of acids and bases in body fluids (very rare). | Upset acid-base balance. |
| POTASSIUM | 775 to 5,625 mg | Bananas, dried fruits, peanut butter, potatoes, orange juice. | With sodium, helps regulate body-fluid balance, transmission of nerve impulses. | Muscular weakness, irritability, irregular heartbeat (rare but may result from prolonged diarrhea or use of diuretics). | High levels of potassium can cause severe cardiac irregularities and can lead to cardiac arrest. |

| | | | | | |
|---|---|---|---|---|---|
| **MAGNESIUM** | 200 to 300 mg | Leafy green vegetables, nuts, soy. | Activator for enzymes that transfer and release energy in the body. | Muscular tremors, twitching and weakness. Deficiency is sometimes seen in people with severe disease, prolonged diarrhea, or alcoholism. | Upset of the calcium-magnesium ratio, leading to impaired nervous-system function. Especially dangerous for people with impaired kidney function. |
| **SULFUR** | | Wheat germ, dried beans, beef, clams. | In every cell as component of several amino acids. | Unknown. | Unknown. |
| **IRON** _TRACE MINERALS_ | 10 to 18 mg | Liver, meat products, egg yolks, shellfish, green leafy vegetables, peas, beans, dried prunes, raisins, apricots, whole-grain and enriched bread and cereal. | Combines with protein to make hemoglobin, the red substance in the blood that carries oxygen from lungs to cells, and myoglobin which stores oxygen in muscles. | Iron-deficiency anemia; pallor of skin, weakness and fatigue, headache, shortness of breath. | Toxic buildup in liver, pancreas, and heart (very rare). |
| **IODINE** | 90 to 150 mcg | Iodized salt, seafoods. | Necessary for normal function of the thyroid gland. | Thyroid enlargement (goiter). Newborns: cretinism. | Could cause poisoning or sensitivity reactions. |

| Nutrient | RDA for Adults and Children Over Four[a] | Some Significant Sources | Some Major Physiological Functions | Some Deficiency Symptoms | Some Overconsumption Symptoms |
| --- | --- | --- | --- | --- | --- |
| ZINC | 10 to 15 mg | Meats, fish, egg yolks, and milk. | Element of the enzymes that through the red blood cells move carbon dioxide from the tissues to the lungs. | Loss of taste and delayed wound healing. Children: growth retardation and delayed sexual maturation. | Gastrointestinal symptoms, such as nausea, vomiting, bleeding, and abdominal pain. Pregnant women: premature labor and stillbirth. |
| COPPER | 2 mg | Organ meats, shellfish, nuts, fruit, dried legumes, raisins, mushrooms. | Occurs as part of important proteins, including enzymes involved in brain and red blood cell function. Also needed for making red blood cells. | Rarely seen in adult humans. Infants: hypochronic anemia with abnormal development of bone; nervous tissue, lungs, and pigmentation of hair. | Gastrointestinal symptoms such as vomiting and diarrhea can occur as a result of eating foods cooked in unlined copper pots. |

| | Amount | Food Sources | Function | Deficiency | Excess |
|---|---|---|---|---|---|
| FLUORIDE | 1 to 4 mg | Fluoridated water and foods cooked in fluoridated water, fish, meat, tea. | Contributes to solid tooth and bone formation, especially in children. May help prevent osteoporosis in older people. | Tooth decay. | Motting of enamel of teeth. |
| CHROMIUM | .03 to .20 mg | Dried brewer's yeast, whole-grain cereal, liver. | With insulin, it is required for utilization of glucose. | Diabeteslike symptoms. | Unknown. |
| SELENIUM | .03 to .20 mg | Seafood, egg yolk, chicken, milk, whole-grain cereals. | Interacts with vitamin E; prevents breakdown of body chemicals. | Unknown in humans. | Unknown. |
| MANGANESE | 1.5 to 5 mg | Bran, coffee, tea, nuts, peas, beans. | Needed for normal tendon and bone structure; part of some enzymes. | Unknown in humans. | Unknown |
| MOLYBDENUM | .06 to .50 mg | Legumes, cereals, dark green vegetables, kidney, liver. | Forms part of the enzyme xantine oxidase. | Unknown in humans. | Loss of copper; joint pain similar to gout. |

Source: Robert J. Weiss, M.D., and Genell Subak-Sharpe, Columbia University School of Public Health *Complete Guide to Health and Well-Being After 50* (New York: Times Books, 1987).

as if, in fact, a normal amount led to the characteristic signs of a deficiency. And other undesirable consequences can be the development of urinary tract problems and blood disorders.

While new information keeps accumulating, there are still vast areas of ignorance about *how the various nutrients interact with each other* and whether there is a crucial difference in how the body reacts to the nutrients when they are metabolized as part of food rather than in the form of capsules. Thus, since extra-large amounts of *any* one nutrient—whether vitamin or mineral—seems to interfere with some other one, many faddish nutrition guides recommend taking supplements of everything. Don't be fooled by claims that a substance is "free of chemicals." No food is free of chemicals because chemicals are what all foods are made of.

Consumers are regularly warned to be alert to advertising and promotion claims that certain foods are "all natural," or that they contain "nothing artificial," or that they are "organically grown." People who have been convinced that the megavitamins they buy in "health-food" stores have greater curative powers because they come from "natural sources" are probably paying higher prices for products that function no differently from their "synthetic" counterparts.

## UNPROVEN CLAIMS FOR NUTRITION THERAPY

Although some doctors and many nutritionists are making these recommendations, the following have been proven by definitive tests for megavitamin and mineral therapy.

- Large doses of vitamin C *have not* proved effective in treating and relieving symptoms of many rheumatic diseases.

- Vitamin B$^6$ *does not* improve the condition of patients with osteoarthritis and rheumatoid arthritis.

- Therapeutic doses of vitamins A and D, most easily available in cod liver oil, are *not* beneficial to patients with rheumatoid arthritis.

- Although patients with rheumatic diseases are likely to suffer from a calcium deficiency, their condition *will not* improve if they take large supplemental doses of calcium.

- When aspirin is combined with copper, it *is not* more effective than cortisone in reducing inflammation. (A recent study—*The New York Times*, February 2, 1988—has actually shown that taking too much copper can interfere with the absorption of zinc and vice versa.)

- Manganese and selenium *have not* been shown to play an important role in rheumatic disease.

## RHEUMATOLOGY RESEARCH

Clinical trials involving vitamins and minerals are an ongoing activity in the scientific community of rheumatologists. Here are some recent conclusions:

- While there is no clinical evidence that vitamin C has therapeutic effects on rheumatoid arthritis, it may have a positive effect on the immune system.

- When patients with rheumatic diseases were treated with copper compounds, some generally favorable results were offset by many adverse effects.

- One study not confirmed by others indicated that there was some improvement in rheumatoid arthritis patients who were treated with zinc.

## PROCEED WITH CAUTION

Since the 1960s there has been an increasing tendency for many men and women dissatisfied with the counsels of conventional medicine to take matters of treatment into their own hands. Those who are wary of taking "medicines" prescribed by a physician because they don't want "all those chemicals in their body" or because "medicines aren't natural and produce bad side effects" should consider that while they may be absolutely right in resenting overmedication, they should also consider that heavy vitamin and mineral doses can be as dangerous as overdoses of any drugs. They can impair body functions, they can lead to physical dependency, and they can throw many metabolic processes into confusion.

If you feel that your arthritis symptoms are held in check or are actually diminishing because of self-prescribed vitamin therapy, *be sure* to have your blood and urine checked regularly. If you are following a special vitamin and mineral regimen prescribed by an accredited nutritionist, such check-ups are likely to be part of the treatment, or should be. If the extra vitamins have been prescribed by your prime-care physician, follow instructions to the letter and don't suddenly decide to discontinue large doses of *anything* without first informing the person who is treating you that you intend to do so.

## HOMEOPATHY

Homeopathy is a system of medical practice based on four principles set down by a nineteenth-century German physician, Dr. Samuel Hahnemann: (1) substances that produce symptoms similar to those experienced by the patient will cure the patient. This is called "the law of similars." (2) Only one dose of the substance is needed. (3) A minimum dose is most potent. (4) In order to attain homeostasis—a relatively stable state of equilibrium within the body—vital forces that are dynamic must also be set in motion by the individual.

Nowadays the National Center for Homeopathy defines the practice as "a system of drug treatment for sick people [not diseases] which is based on the Law of Similars, the minimum dose and the single remedy proven on human beings."

While homeopathic practitioners do not claim to cure diseases in cases of physical malformation, tissue damage, advanced cancer, or cases where major surgery is indicated, supporters claim that homeopathic methods can be used successfully for most reversible illnesses and many acute infections. However, because the practitioners treat not a specific disease but rather a set of symptoms, they do not claim to have any one single treatment for arthritis or related conditions.

If you should embark on a homeopathic treatment program for a rheumatic disorder, you'll probably be given a small dose of something from the approved pharmacopoeia that will temporarily increase (or aggravate) your joint inflammation according to the principle "let like be cured by like." Homeopathic remedies are often selected from "natural" substances such as plants and minerals. As a patient in this procedure, you'll be expected to follow instructions with care and not disturb the balances that the practitioner is attempting to achieve. While faith and cooperation are considered indispensable to effective treatment, a dash of healthy skepticism is in order if the treatment turns out to involve several substances rather than the One and Only supposedly indicated for your particular symptoms.

Additional information about homeopathy and its practitioners is available from the

National Center for Homeopathy
1500 Massachusetts Avenue NW
Washington, DC 20005
202-223-6182

## NATUROPATHY

Unlike homeopathy, which, in undertaking to treat a chronic condition like arthritis, makes a list of "strong" symptoms and then searches for the drug that would appear to cause the same symptoms, naturopathic practitioners use a more eclectic approach. Taking what they consider to be a holistic view of the patient, they describe themselves as treating disease and restoring health by investigating the patient's hereditary, biological, and environmental problems. After establishing a detailed profile of the individual through various diagnostic tests, they set up a treatment that draws on nutrition, herbal medicine, homeopathy, exercise, acupuncture, hydrotherapy, and counseling. They place special emphasis on sunbathing, steam baths, exercise, and diet, and prohibit the use of salt and stimulants. They believe strongly in the healing powers of nature, and in their literature they assert that "the naturopathic approach to health care can prevent minor illness from developing into more serious or chronic degenerative diseases."

Naturopathic practitioners are not medical doctors and the credentials they do have are highly suspect in many quarters. The "degree" of N.D., which stands for Doctor of Naturopathy, is conferred on them by either one of two colleges of Naturopathic medicine in the United States. One is in Seattle, Washington, the other in Portland, Oregon. Practitioners with an N.D. degree are licensed to practice medicine in six states only: Arizona, Arkansas, Connecticut, Hawaii, Oregon, and Washington. Naturopathic "healers'" and holistic practitioners without credentials are to be found nationwide.

Additional information is available from the

American Association of Naturopathic Physicians
P.O. Box 33046
Portland, Oregon 97233
503-255-4863

## HYDROTHERAPY

"Taking the waters," both internally and externally, is an old tradition that continues to be more honored nowadays in Europe than in the United States. Many Romans, like their ancient ancestors, still praise the curative powers of nearby mineral springs so rich in sulfur that you have to hold your nose when you approach them. The town of Spa in Belgium was so popular for several centuries that it became the generic term for all watering places; the waters of Evian, not to mention Perrier, are profitably bottled and distributed worldwide. And while you're likely to find more New Yorkers in Saratoga Springs for the horse racing than for the "cure," there's a growing interest among people with arthritis in the hydrotherapy offered as a special feature by health spas in the States and in Mexico.

As anyone with a rheumatic condition knows, water plays an important part in easing inflammation and, in many cases, slowing down and possibly halting the degenerative process of joint tissues. Advocates of hydrotherapy point to the many procedures based on water: wrapping swollen joints in alternating hot and cold compresses; exercising regularly when partially submerged in a warm bath; directional underwater "massaging" by a powerful stream of water.

## LOCAL SOURCES

While it's true that some of the more esoteric types of hydrotherapy such as mud baths and salt rubs are available only at vacation spas, other types, such as Turkish baths and saunas, are a routine aspect of many local health-club memberships. And practically all provide the use of a good-sized swimming pool for those indispensable underwater workouts.

It's a good idea to speak to your doctor about how to get optimum benefits from various forms of hydrotherapy on a regular basis. Also, find out whether to invest in one of those electrically controlled felt-surfaced pads that provide wet heat. These pads (trade name Thermaphore) are equipped with temperature regulators, and when you own one there's no longer any need to go through the process of putting a heavy towel in hot water and wringing it out so that you can take it to bed with you to ease joint pain.

## CELLULAR THERAPY

An aura of mystery surrounds the treatment known as *cellular therapy*, which is practiced by a number of posh clinics in Switzerland. Many important personages have claimed that this treatment has not only rejuvenated internal organs and tissues but has also brought about a significant improvement in their mobility, previously hampered by arthritis.

In cellular therapy, using unborn lambs as their source, clinicians harvest living cells from the fetuses' various organs—

kidneys, stomach, liver, skeleton, and so forth. (The skeleton in all unborn animals, including humans, is made of cartilage, which eventually hardens into bone.) These extracted cells are grouped into categories and are then injected into the patient's muscles on the theory that the cells will produce a regeneration of the diseased tissues by eventually finding their way to the part of the body for which they are designated.

Cellular therapy has its enthusiastic supporters. In the scientific community it has been suggested that if this therapy works at all, it may be because the injections reinforce the genetic information within the degenerated tissues, stimulating them to renew themselves.

Detailed information about cellular therapy is unavailable in this country because this type of treatment is illegal in the United States.

## LASERS

Because light interacts with living tissue, a new field has developed called *photomedicine,* which involves the teamwork of several different specialists. During the nineteenth century the discovery of ultraviolet light (the radiation located beyond the visible spectrum at its violet end) was followed by the discovery that it could be used as a deadly weapon against bacteria. Before the development of medicines that proved to be more effective, it was used as a treatment for tuberculosis of the skin. Until vitamin D deficiency was found to be the specific cause of rickets, exposure to sunlight or artificial ultraviolet light was the accepted way to prevent or even halt the progress of this once-widespread bone disease. Nowadays UV light is the treatment of choice for psoriasis and may prove to be a useful tool in the treatment of certain types of cancer.

The most recent development in photomedicine is the use of lasers. Lasers are highly concentrated light beams that can be adjusted to specific wavelengths—from ultraviolet to visible to infrared parts of the spectrum. It seems almost inconceivable that these beams, which are controlled so that they can be flashed on for very brief periods, are powerful enough to cut through diamonds. They can convey enough heat to cauterize bleeding tissue, and because their focus can be directed to an almost infinitesimal point, they can zero in on diseased tissue and destroy it with greater precision than the steadiest hand holding the tinest surgical knife.

Recently many different kinds of lasers have been developed for use in the communications industry and by the military. Their use in eye surgery has become standard practice. Still in the experimental state is their use in cleaning out the accumulated plaque within blood vessels and in destroying diseased cells in cervical cancer.

While some doctors have reported benefits of laser irradiation for patients with rheumatoid arthritis, most rheumatologists are included to wait for the results of further experimentation. In the meantime there are reports that venturesome patients have bought units intended for use in veterinary medicine and tried them on their backs, feet, hands, and other badly afflicted joints. Some claimed beneficial results.

One controlled study showed no benefits when compared with placebo laser treatment. But laser technology applied to medical science is in its infancy and may yet prove to be an effective treatment for rheumatic diseases.

Some of the treatments described in this chapter have been helpful to some arthritis patients. In a number of cases they have been especially helpful when combined with conventional medical and surgical treatment. For someone with mild aches and pains, there's little risk in accepting the recommendations of a herbalist or a holistic practitioner with scant credentials. But the risk is serious for anyone with a rheumatic disease, which, if properly and properly diagnosed, can be effectively treated by conventional medicine and/or surgery before it does further damage. In these cases accurate diagnosis may be based on laboratory techniques and expensive equipment available only to qualified physicians with hospital connections.

## PSYCHOLOGICAL TREATMENTS

While the role played by brain/mind activities in altering the disease *process* continues to be somewhat controversial, the techniques associated with altering states of consciousness are increasingly incorporated into pain therapy. These techniques are discussed in Chapter Nine.

## A POSTSCRIPT ON QUACKERY

According to the U.S. Food and Drug Administration, "Health fraud or quackery robs Americans of an estimated $10 billion annually through worthless and often harmful products," and of this amount, congressional studies estimate that in a recent year over $2 billion was spent by arthritis sufferers on phony remedies, procedures, and gadgets.

Because of the erratic nature of the symptoms of many rheumatic diseases, extravagant claims can be made for this or that quack "cure" if its use happens to coincide with one of the long periods of remission that characterize the unpredictability of many cases. Also, because joint diseases are responsive to treatment from the outside, such as heat, water, and massage, it is easy to prey on the gullible about the "magic" powers of such devices as "inductoscopes" and "vitalators."

The full range of quack cures for arthritis may be lacking in validity, but it does show lots of imagination. Here's a sampling: sitting in an inactive uranium mine; taping nickels to your legs; putting zinc heels on your shoes; wearing copper bracelets; being injected with everything from bee venom to olive oil, and rubbing yourself with the industrial solvent dimethyl sulfoxide (DMSO). This latter, promoted as a healing ointment, is still legally available in some "health-food" stores in spite of continued warnings by the FDA about its dangerous side effects.

Even though you may be impatient with conventional treatment and are exploring alternative ways to cope with arthritis, be alert to unscrupulous promoters who make millions by exploiting other people's misery. A report issued by the Council of Better Business Bureaus called "Arthritis: Quackery and Unproven Remedies" contains the following warnings:

- Be wary of "cures" or "guaranteed cures."

- Look for certain key words. "Breakthrough," "secret," "exclusive," or "special" are not scientific words and often appear for promotions of quack products. Cures for serious medical problems are not usually available through the mails.

- Be cautious if immediate, complete relief of undiagnosed pain is guaranteed.

- Be cautious of vaguely worded testimonials that cannot be verified. Also, an ethical health practitioner is not likely to advertise accomplishments about miracles performed on famous people. Testimonials should not serve as a substitute for scientific proof of a product's efficacy.

- Be wary of any special diet or nutrition treatment program promoted as a cure. Research scientists have not found any foods or nutrients that cause arthritis or make it better or worse (except that some foods have a role in triggering gout, a form of arthritis).

- Be wary of any group promoting distrust, e.g., "Your family physician doesn't know about this," "Don't listen to the Food and Drug Administration," etc.

- Watch out for any advertisements that claim Food and Drug Administration (FDA) approval. Federal law does not permit the mention of the FDA or the U.S. Food and Drug Administration in any way that suggests marketing approval for any drug or medical device.

- Beware of claims that a product offered as a cure for arthritis is also a cure for other serious health problems.

- If you have questions about an advertised product, investigate the company and the product by checking with your nearest FDA office and Better Business Bureau *before* buying.

- Be wary of health remedies sold door-to-door by peddlers or self-proclaimed health advisers who sell their product at public lectures, traveling from town to town. High-pressure sales tactics and one-time-only deals are clues that something is wrong.

A complete five-page report is available from your local Better Business Bureau, or write to the

Council of Better Business Bureaus, Inc.
4200 Wilson Blvd.
Arlington, VA 22073

Enclose a self-addressed, stamped business envelope with your request.


# A FEW WORDS ABOUT THE FUTURE

Each year brings new and improved ways of treating arthritis and of helping you cope with it more effectively. Remarkable achievements in the use of arthroscopy and in the techniques of joint replacements have occurred recently. Prime-care doctors marvel at the newfound mobility of their previously disabled patients when they leave their wheelchairs behind, thanks to prosthetic knees and hips.

Surgical procedures are constantly being refined: computer science is playing an increasingly important role in the creation of prosthetic joints individually designed for each recipient, and the science of robotics is advancing the precision with which operations on the joints can be performed.

At the Massachusetts Institute of Technology, weight distribution is a special area of research. Engineers with expertise in the science of stresses and strains join with specialists in biomechanics to achieve a better understanding of how human joints fit together—and the result for arthritis patients is better strengthening exercises, self-help devices, and rehabilitation equipment for improving mobility and reducing pain.

The same institution has been conducting experiments that yield information about the pressures to which hip cartilage is subjected. In the course of this research it has been discovered that peak pressures occur not when you're standing or walking, or even jogging, but when you get up from a chair. This information is leading not only to special new chair designs but is also a useful guide in the design of prosthetic hip joints, strengthening them at specific weight-bearing points.

## DRUGS

Pharmaceutical companies are testing more than 200 drugs in the nonsteroidal (NSAID) and disease-modifying (DMARD) categories, with the conviction that these tests will soon yield anti-rheumatic medications superior in effectiveness to anything now available. They are also exploring the ways in which two anti-cancer drugs—interferon and interleuken—can be used to help people with severe rheumatoid arthritis.

The future may bring a drug capable of altering a key metabolic process in somewhat the same way that drugs control gout. It is known that when joints are used, they release enzymes that digest cartilage at the same time that healthy cartilage keeps repairing the damage. Biochemists are working on ways either of blocking the enzyme or stimulating the cartilage so that a protective balance can be achieved between the two processes.

The connection between the nervous system and the inflammatory response is yielding a new application of a powerful drug now in use only for life-threatening high blood pressure. The observation that stroke victims rarely develop arthritis on the side of the body impaired by the stroke has led to the belief that the same drug (guanethidine) that blocks the action of the sympathetic nervous system might be effective in reducing inflammation. In the experimental cases where it has been tried, patients have reported a decrease in pain and an increase in joint strength.

## OTHER PROMISING AREAS

Geneticists are trying to find out why people who have inherited a tendency to develop arthritis actually do develop it. When they discover what triggers the onset they expect to be able to suppress it.

The arthritis symptoms of Lyme disease have led to an increased interest in the theory that rheumatoid arthritis is in fact an infectious disease, one in which the rubella (German measles) virus and the Epstein-Barr (monoculeosis and herpes) virus are specifically implicated. If and when this should prove true, it should theoretically be possible to develop a vaccine as an effective form of therapy.

A new procedure whose long-term results may bring long periods of relief to those with rheumatoid arthritis consists of injecting a radioactive isotope directly into the damaged joint. The injection cauterizes the diseased matter without affecting the surrounding healthy tissue, and by removing it, the inflammation is successfully arrested.

## AS FOR THE PRESENT

Whether your arthritis problems are no more than a minor nuisance or they are indeed a major concern; remember that although there's no definite cure, there's a wide range of treatments. Be realistic in your expectations, and establish a productive working partnership with your doctor. Self-reliance goes with self-respect, but ask for help from family members, professional counselors, and support groups when you need it. Make every effort to maintain normal relationships and seek out those friends and activities that cheer you up. And, above all, don't forget that you're not only a patient—you're a person with a full, gratifying life to live!

# GLOSSARY

*acetaminophen* (Tylenol, Anacin-3, Datril) a medicine that reduces pain and fever but does not counteract inflammation

*acupuncture* an ancient Chinese therapy in which certain points on the body's surface are stimulated by rotating fine needles in order to influence other parts of the body.

*acute* having a brief and usually severe course

*aerobics* exercises whose purpose is the improvement of respiratory and circulatory efficiency by increasing oxygen consumption

*allopurinol* a drug used in the treatment of gout to increase the secretion of uric acid

*analgesic* causing relief of pain; also the agent that does so

*ankylosing spondylitis* inflammation of the spinal vertebrae that can cause them to grow together

*antigen* a substance capable of stimulating the immune system

*arthralgia* pain in a joint

*arthrocentesis* the insertion of a hollow needle into a joint for the purpose of withdrawing a sample of synovial fluid

*arthrodesis* immobilizing the bones of a joint so that the surfaces become fused; a surgical procedure also known as artificial ankylosis

*arthropathy* any disease of a joint

*arthroplasty* plastic surgery of a joint

*arthroscopy* examination of the interior of a joint through a special surgical instrument

*autoimmune* relating to the antibodies that attack the very tissues that they have been produced to protect

*biofeedback* a process whereby a person is given auditory or visual information concerning such bodily activities as heartbeat or brain waves for the purpose of consciously controlling them

*Bouchard's nodes* bony growths on the middle joints of the fingers, usually a symptom of degenerative joint disease

*bursa* a fluid-filled pouch-like cavity situated in parts of a joint or the connective tissue to help reduce friction and absorb shock

*bursitis* inflammation of a bursa

*carpal tunnel syndrome* inflammation of the tendons of the wrist, causing the tunnel of bones and ligaments in the wrist to narrow, thereby pinching the nerves that reach the fingers and the muscle at the base of the thumb

*cartilage* strong elastic tissue that serves as a shock absorber at the ends of bones

*CAT scan* see *computed tomography*

*chiropractic* a system of treatment based on the belief that manipulation of skeletal components, especially of the spine, can restore the health of the nervous system

*chondrocyte* a cartilage cell

*chondromalacia patellae* softening of the cartilage that cushions the kneecap

*chondroplasty* plastic surgery for the purpose of repairing damaged cartilage

*chronic* lasting over a long period, usually throughout a lifetime

*colchicine* a drug derived from a plant and used for centuries to suppress the pain of a gout attack

*collagen* a protein component of bones and connective tissue that is transformed into gelatin when boiled

*computed tomography;* also *computed axial tomography* a radiographic procedure 100 times more sensitive than X ray that creates a three-dimensional image of a body structure by superimposing its various layers into a composite of differing intensities

*connective tissue* ligaments, tendons, and muscles that bend and support bones

*corticosteroids* any of the steroids produced by the adrenal cortex; also their synthetic analogs

*cortisone* a corticosteroid used sparingly in the treatment of arthritis

*cyst* an abnormal growth in the form of a membrane-enclosed sac that develops within or on a body structure

*degenerative joint disease* a form of arthritis usually associated with aging; formerly called osteoarthritis

*DMARDs* disease-modifying anti-rheumatic drugs; a category of powerful medications thought to control the destructive process of rheumatoid arthritis

*dysplasia* abnormal growth or development of a body structure; in arthritis, faulty relationship between the bones in a joint, increasing the likelihood of inflammation

*femur* (adj. *femoral*) thighbone

*fibrositis* pain and inflammation in the connective tissues, i.e., muscles, ligaments, and tendons; sometimes called *muscle rheumatism*

*flare; flare-up* the sudden reappearance or intensification of symptoms

*fungal arthritis* development of arthritis symptoms secondary to a systemic fungal infection

*ganglion* a small cyst-like tumor attached to a joint membrane

*genetic marker* a specific tissue type passed down through the genes from one generation to the next; a link has been established between certain genetic markers and certain rheumatic diseases

*gonococcal arthritis* development of arthritis symptoms secondary to gonorrhea infection

*gout* a form of arthritis in which the crystals from excessive uric acid in the blood collect and settle in the joint space, usually of the big toe, causing acute pain and inflammation

*Heberden's nodes* bony growths on the finger joints just below the nails; a characteristic of degenerative joint disease, especially in women

*hydrotherapy* the use of water in treating disease

*ibuprofen* (Motrin, Rufen by prescription; Advil, Nuprin nonprescription) a nonsteroidal anti-inflammatory drug (NSAID)

*idiopathic* not traceable to any cause; appearing to arise spontaneously

*immune system* the battery of defenses with which the body protects itself against injury and disease

*immunosuppressant drugs* medication that attempts to stop or slow the abnormal behavior of the immune system when it engages in the destruction instead of the protection of the body's tissues

*indomethacin* (Indocin) a nonsteroidal anti-inflammatory drug (NSAID)

*infectious arthritis* arthritis that results from a bacterial, viral, or fungal infection

*inflammation* a condition of redness, heat, swelling, and pain that develops when the body's defenses begin to ward off the effects of injury or infection; in arthritis, however, inflammation is part of the disease rather than a transitional state

*joint* any part of the body where two bones come together

*juvenile arthritis* the inclusive term for various kinds of arthritis that begin in childhood

*joint fluid* see *synovial fluid*

*laser therapy* the use of extremely high-powered radiologic beams for treatment by irradiation of various disorders; still largely experimental

*ligament* a tough cordlike structure that connects one bone to another

*lumbrosacral* relating to the lower back

*lupus* see *systemic lupus erythematosus*

*Lyme disease* a multiphased systemic bacterial disease caused by the bite of a tick that infests deer. If not treated correctly and promptly with heavy doses of antibiotics, severe joint inflammation may be an eventual result

*magnetic resonance imaging* a noninvasive diagnostic procedure that provides extremely bright, high-contrast, images of body tissues

*methotrexate* a disease-modifying anti-rheumatic drug (DMARD) used with some success to slow down the destructive process of rheumatoid arthritis

*mycoplasma arthritis* a secondary arthritis following infection with microorganisms that may cause a type of pneumonia. The mycoplasma organisms are intermediate between bacteria and viruses; tetracycline is the effective treatment

*naproxen* (Naprosyn) a nonsteroidal anti-inflammatory drug (NSAID)

*National Institute for Arthritis, Musculoskeletal and Skin Diseases* a recently formed research institute, part of the National Institutes of Health (NIH) under the jurisdiction of the United States Department of Health and Human Services

*nonsteroidal anti-inflammatory drug* (NSAID) any of a gorup of medicines that relieve pain and control inflammation

*NSAIDs* see above

*orthotics* the use of supports, braces, splints, and the like in the treatment of weak or nonfunctional muscles

*osteitis deformans* see *Paget's disease*

*osteoarthritis* a distinction is now made between *degenerative joint disease* (q.v.) and other forms of the chronic joint disease that are essentially non-inflammatory

*osteomalacia* a softening of the bones in adults, similar to rickets in children, and not to be confused with *osteoporosis* (q.v.)

*osteomyelitis* inflammation of the bone caused by infection

*osteopathy* medical practice based on the principle that diseases result essentially from faulty alignment of musculoskeletal components. Treatment consists of corrective manipulation supplemented when necessary by medicine and surgery

*osteoporosis* decrease in bone mass and density leading to some skeletal deformity and increased bone fragility. Like degenerative joint disease, osteoporosis is a factor of aging, but there is no causal relationship between the two conditions

*Paget's disease* a chronic disorder characterized by the weakening, enlargement, and deformation of bones; also called *osteitis deformans*

*patella*  the kneecap

*penicillamine* (Cuprimine, Depen)  a powerful anti-inflammatory drug that, because of its serious side effects, requires close monitoring

*phenylbutazone* (Butazolidin)  one of the earliest nonsteroidal anti-inflammatory drugs, now rarely used because of negative side effects

*physiatrist*  a physician with an M.D. degree who specializes in physical medicine and rehabilitation

*physical therapy*  nonmedical nonsurgical treatment based on the use of exercise, massage, heat, light, water, electricity, and the like

*piroxicam* (Feldene)  one of the preferred nonsteroidal anti-inflammatory drugs taken only once a day

*poststreptococcal arthritis*  joint inflammation following rheumatic fever or other streptococcus infection for which treatment is delayed

*prednisone* (Deltasone)  an anti-inflammatory drug analogous to cortisone

*probencid* (Benemid)  a drug used in the treatment of gout

*prostaglandins*  hormone-like natural substances that perform many functions, only some of which are understood: stimulation of muscle contraction, lowering of blood pressure, influence on hormonal processes. Inhibiting the action of some prostaglandins appears to be a positive effect of several of the anti-inflammatory drugs

*prothesis*  an artificial replacement for a missing part of the body for functional and/or esthetic reasons

*pseudogout*  joint inflammation caused by crystal deposits of calcium pyrophosphate dihydrate (CPPD). Although any joint may be affected, the likeliest site is the knee. Pseudogout is treated effectively with nonsteroidial anti-inflammatory drugs.

*psoriatic arthritis*  a form of arthritis related to and accompanying the skin disease psoriasis. Treatment is similar to that for rheumatoid arthritis

*rehabilitation*  the use of a broad range of treatments to reestablish normal form and function to parts of the body damaged by injury or disease; also the restoration of an individual's capabilities for maximum competence in all possible spheres of normal life following illness, injury, substance abuse, etc.

*Reiter's syndrome* a type of arthritis precipitated by infection of the gastrointestinal or genitourinary tract; other associated conditions include conjunctivitis and oral ulcers. The joint involvement, usually of the knees and ankles, usually begins two to six weeks after the onset of the original infection. Another characteristic is the conspicuous swelling of fingers and toes, called *sausage digits.* Nonsteroidal anti-inflammatory drugs are the preferred treatment.

*remission* the diminishing or abatement of disease symptoms; also, the period during which the symptoms are gone

*Reye's syndrome* a life-threatening disease, especially of childhood, associated with the use of aspirin for fever occurring during such viral infections as chicken pox and the flu

*rheumatic diseases* a group of diseases affecting ligaments, tendons, muscles, joints, as well as other parts of the body

*rheumatic fever* an acute disease of childhood and adolescence characterized by fever, joint inflammation, and coronary involvement. The pains in and around the joints used to be referred to as "growing pains"; when ignored or not promptly treated by rest and anti-inflammatory drugs, the result can be irreversible damage to heart valves

*rheumatoid arthritis* a usually chronic disease affecting the entire system but especially characterized by pain, stiffness, swelling, inflammation, and, in some cases, destruction of joints

*rheumatologist* a medical doctor who specializes in the diagnosis and treatment of rheumatic diseases

*salicylic acid* the active ingredient in aspirin and similar drugs used to reduce pain and fever and especially in the treatment of arthritis as an anti-inflammatory agent

*scleroderma* a chronic disease characterized by the shrinking and hardening of the connective tissues in various parts of the body including the skin

*SLE* see *systemic lupus erythematosus*

*steroid* any of a group of compounds sharing the same chemical composition; cholesterol, progesterone, and cortisone are members of this group

*subluxation* a partial or total dislocation of a joint

*sulindac (Clinoril)* a nonsteroidal anti-inflammatory drug

*synovectomy* surgical removal of the synovial membrane

*synovial fluid* transparent substance, similar to eggwhite, secreted by the synovial membrane and contained in the cavities of joints as well as in bursae and tendon sheaths

*synovial membrane* the thin layer of tissue that lines the cavity in which a joint is contained

*systemic disease* a disease that affects many parts of the body

*systemic lupus erythematosus* a rheumatic disease that affects the skin, muscles, and joints, and, in many cases, various internal organs

*tendinitis* inflammation of a tendon

*tendon* a tough band of tissue that connects muscle to bone

*tenosynovitis* inflammation of the membranous sheath that covers a tendon

*TENS* see *transcutaneous electrical nerve stimulation*

*tick* any of a large group of bloodsucking parasites that live on warm-blooded vertebrates and whose bite transmits infectious diseases to humans; Rocky Mountain fever and Lyme disease are tick-borne

*tolmetin* (Tolectin) a nonsteroidal anti-inflammatory drug

*transcutaneous electrical nerve stimulation (TENS)* a small battery-operated device that, through electrodes placed on the skin at special trigger points, stimulates the nerves that block out pain when it is turned on by the user

# APPENDIX:
## Useful Addresses

For information about local groups, referrals, pamphlets, special services, etc.:

The Arthritis Foundation, P.O. Box 19000, Atlanta, Georgia 30306

For information about self-help groups in your area for you and your family:

The National Self-Help Clearing House, 25 West 43rd Street, New York, N.Y. 10036

For catalogs of special merchandise:

Enrichments, Inc., 145 Tower Drive, P.O. Box 579, Hinsdale, Illinois 60521

Dr. Leonards' Health Care Catalogue, 74-20th Street, Brooklyn, N.Y. 11232

For information about accredited pain treatment centers in your area:

The Commission on Accreditation of Rehabilitation Facilities 2500 N. Pantano Road, Tucson, Arizona, 85715

The American Pain Society, 1615 L Street NW, Suite 925, Washington, D.C. 20036

The Committee on Pain Therapy and Acupuncture, American Society of Anesthesiologists, 515 Busse Highway, Park Ridge, Illinois 60068

For information about home-care agencies and services in your area:
  National Association for Home Care, 519 C Street NE, Washington, D.C. 20002

For information about your prescription medicines, request the free pamphlet:
  Rx Drugs, Dept. 62, Pueblo, Colorado 81009

For information about physical therapists in your area:
  American Physical Therapy Association, 1156 15th Street NW, Washington, D.C. 20005

For information about the Well Spouse Foundation:
  Jeanne Watral, P.O. Box 58022, Pittsburgh, Pennsylvania 15209

For information and referral about systemic lupus erythematosus:
  Lupus Foundation of America, 119-21A Olive Blvd., St. Louis, Missouri 63141

For referral to an osteopathic practitioner in your area:
  National Board of Osteopathic Medical Examiners, 2700 River Road, Suite 407, Des Plaines, Illinois 60018

For information about other practitioners:
  Society for Clinical and Experimental Hypnosis, 129A Kings Park Drive, Liverpool, N.Y. 13088
  National Center for Homeopathy, 1500 Massachusetts Avenue NW, Washington, D.C. 20005
  American Association of Natureopathic Physicians, P.O. Box 33046, Portland, Oregon 97233

For reporting frauds, false advertising, and the like:
  Council of Better Business Bureaus, Inc., 4200 Wilson Blvd, Arlington, Virginia 22073

# INDEX

Helene MacLean has been writing about medical and health topics for more than twenty years. She is the editor of *Everywoman's Health: A Complete Guide to Body and Mind* (fourth edition) and of *Women's Occupational Health Resource Center News*. Her most recent book is *Caring for Your Parents* (Doubleday). She lives and works in New York City.